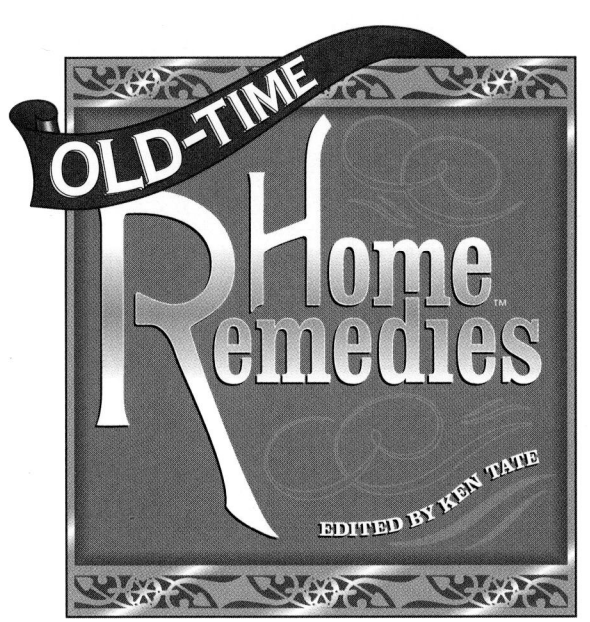

OLD-TIME

Home Remedies™

EDITED BY KEN TATE

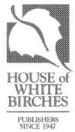

HOUSE of
WHITE
BIRCHES

PUBLISHERS
SINCE 1947

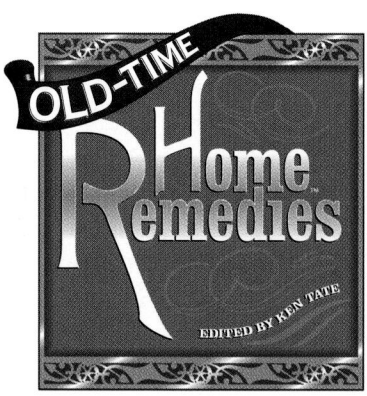

OLD-TIME Home Remedies

EDITED BY KEN TATE

Copyright © 1998 House of White Birches, Berne, Indiana 46711

Editors: Ken and Janice Tate
Copy Editor: Läna Schurb
Associate Editor: Barb Sprunger

Production Manager: Vicki Macy
Creative Coordinator: Shaun Venish
Design/Production Artist: Becky Sarasin
Traffic Coordinator: Sandra Beres
Production Assistants: Shirley Blalock, Dana Brotherton,
Carol Dailey, Cheryl Lynch, Chad Tate

Publishers: Carl H. Muselman, Arthur K. Muselman
Chief Executive Officer: John Robinson
Marketing Director: Scott Moss
Editorial Director: Vivian Rothe
Production Director: Scott Smith

Printed in the United States of America
First Printing: 1998
Library of Congress Number: 97-72868
ISBN: 1-882138-30-9

Dear Friends of the Good Old Days,

"You can't teach an old dog new tricks." Never has that old saying applied more to me than in the area of my health. I grew up in an area and an era when the doctor was literally the last person you would see when you were sick. The first was Mama; if she couldn't handle the situation, Grandma was called in, followed by the granny woman up the road about a quarter-mile. Finally, if all else failed, Doc Evans was contacted.

Today—I have to admit it—I still tend to make the doctor's office the court of last resort. Janice and I have a small herb garden in which we grow everything from comfrey to garlic to peppermint. We cut sassafras roots in the late winter and drink tea from it the remainder of the season to ward off colds and other maladies. I take cayenne to help keep my blood pressure down, and Janice still fixes me a hot cup of camomile tea if my stomach acts up. (I have never taken an drugstore antacid in my life.) The only thing I haven't been able to handle pretty much on my own has been my eyesight.

It is hard to change from the habits of self-dependency taught by generations of trial and error. The tricks of modern medicine are more appropriate to teach a generation younger than me.

When Janice and I conceived this book, we wanted to make it a collection of stories that would run the gamut from actual remedy recipes to stories of how they were used back in the Good Old Days. We hope this look back at the way it was before hospitals, specialists and organ transplants will bring you knowledge and understanding, laughter and tears. Who knows? Maybe this old dog can help bring a younger generation some old tricks from the medicine bag of *Old-Time Home Remedies*.

Sincerely,

Ken Tate

Editor

Contents

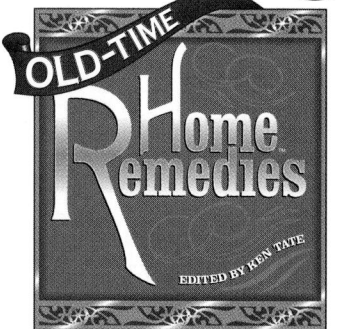

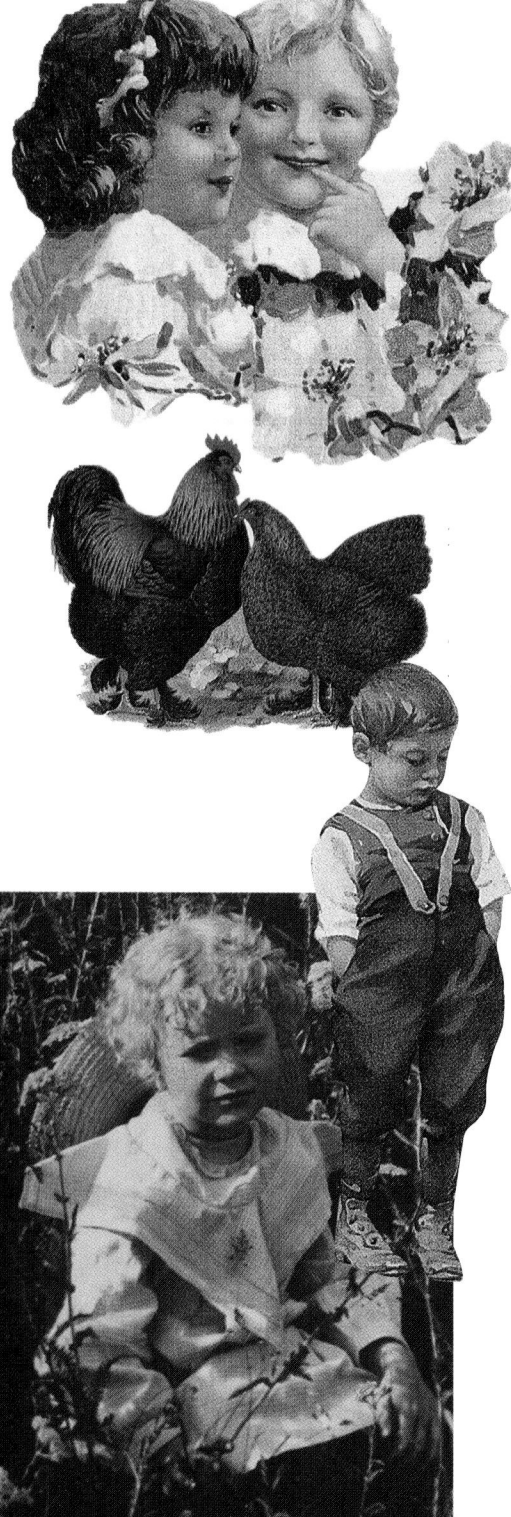

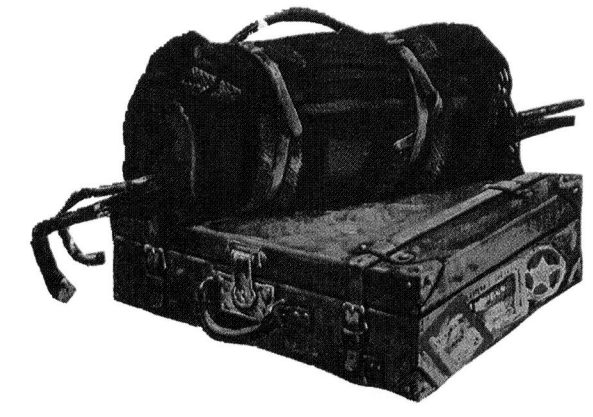

Chapter 4——Miracles or Myths?

Chapter 5——Country Doctors, a Family Friend

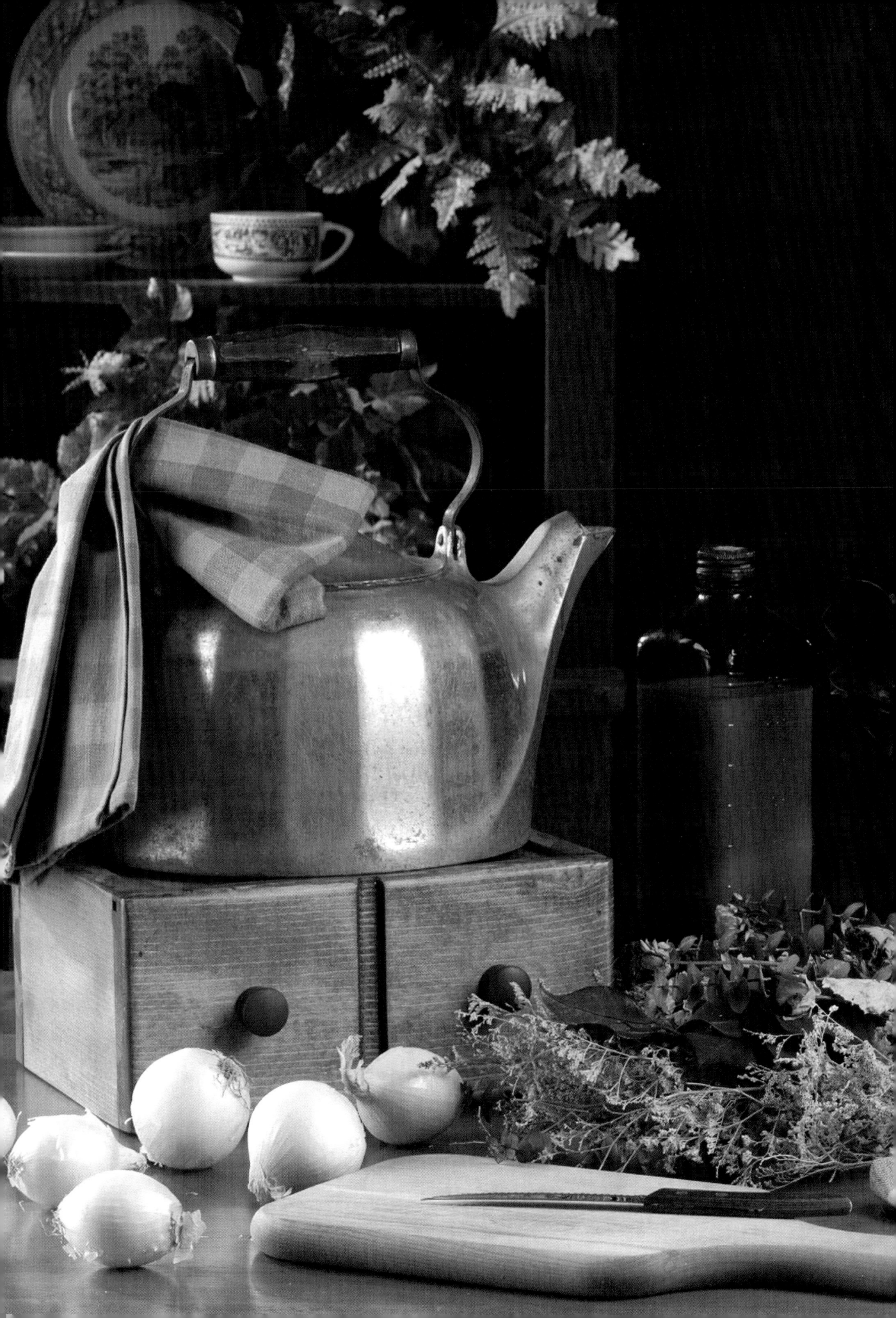

Chapter 1

WONDER OF HERBS

My childhood home was 10 miles from the nearest town, on a hilltop in the Ozark Mountains of southern Missouri. While there was a doctor in town—Doc Evans—we country kids rarely saw him unless it was some type of emergency. To offset that deficiency of city doctoring, Mama always had one remedy or another from her country doctoring bag of tricks.

At one time or another she or Grandma—Mama's medical tutor—tried just about every herb, poultice, tea and tincture on us kids. Sometimes we wondered which was worse, the disease or the cure. Today, whenever I think of Mama's attempts to keep us healthy or get us well, I remember the love and compassion she put with every cure. These stories and recipes from herbal history and lore will remind you of the days when medicine was in the garden and woods rather than in the bottle and pill.

—*Ken Tate*

Whatever Happened to Asafetida?

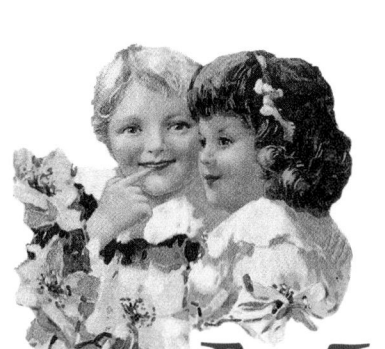

By Sarah Fitzjarrald

My mother's system of preventive health care preceded the establishment of city and county health departments by two full decades and followed not too far behind the organization of the American Medical Association.

When "God bestowed upon her" (her expression) three children—twin girls and a boy—she made a decision early on to keep the kids healthy and out from underfoot, a decision with which my father concurred. They felt it was much better than getting us hooked on too much tender loving care, and having us whining around the house to be waited on hand and foot.

Mother's methods seldom approached the heroic but they were effective. At the first "I don't feel so good," she felt the offender's forehead and ordered him to stick out his tongue. She could tell in a split second whether it was the threat of a math test at school or a real case of the blahs, but her response was always the same. Out came the bottle of Dr. Caldwell's Syrup of Pepsin and the suggestion that the patient go to bed for awhile. More often than not, just the appearance of Dr. Caldwell effected an instant cure. His potion wasn't that bad, but the aftermath was devastating.

We heard stories from some of our classmates that going to bed at their house wasn't all that bad. In fact, some of them got to loll around and read books, and their mothers brought them orange juice and store-bought canned soup!

Going to bed at our house was Dullsville. We couldn't read lying down, and besides, "You shouldn't strain your eyes if you are coming down with measles or mumps, or, God forbid, diphtheria."

Mother wasn't all that gone on orange juice, either. We got glasses and glasses of water to help the Syrup of Pepsin "clean the poison out of your system." We did get a can (or cans) of store-bought soup, but our illnesses seldom lasted through more than two cans at most, and the soup was more for Mother's convenience than ours. She wasn't about to change her mind about what to have for dinner, and she usually managed to fix something which smelled delicious for dessert—for the rest of the family. But Mother wasn't deliberately cruel. After a usually speedy

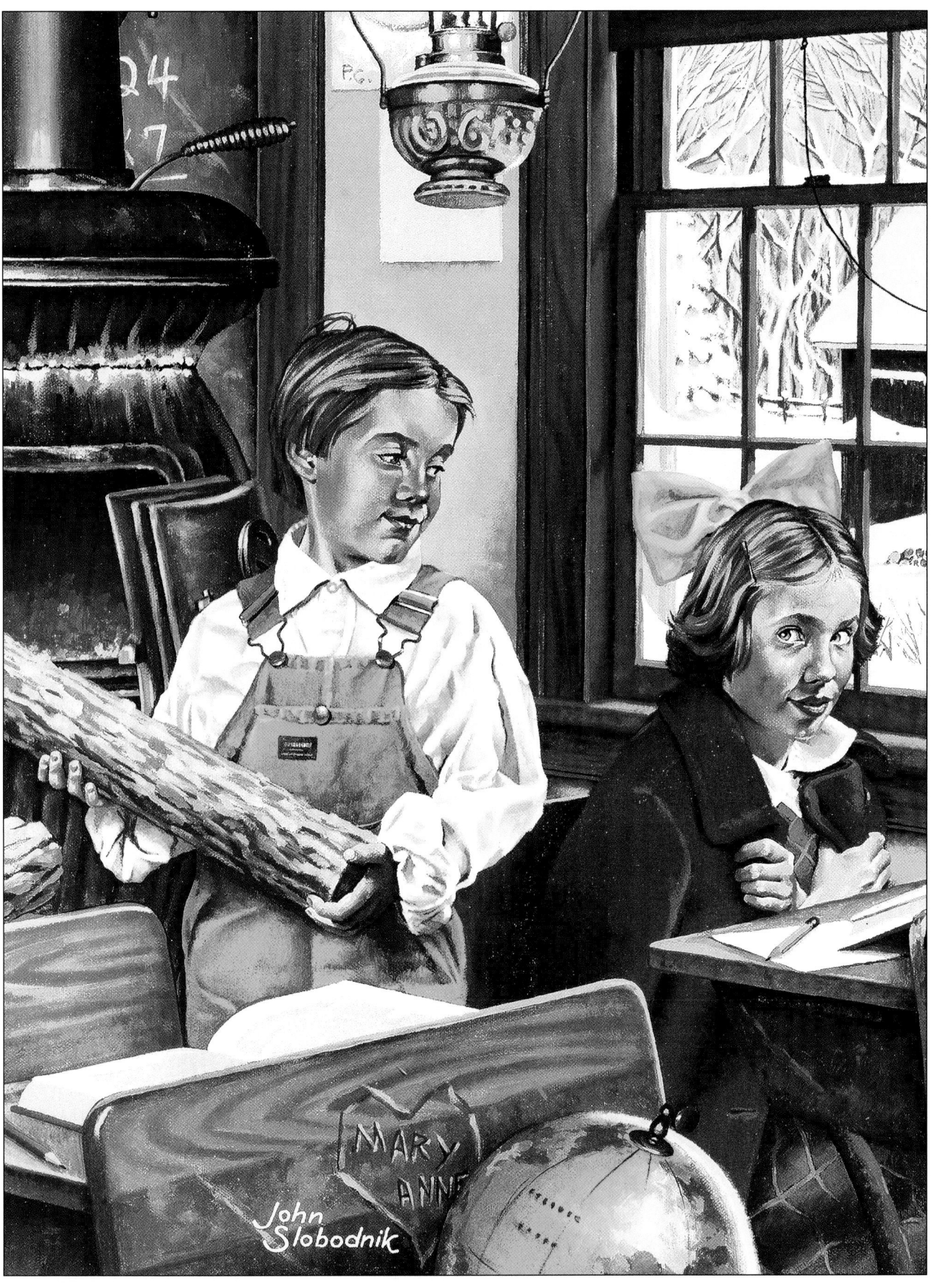

recovery we always found that she had saved us a piece of apple pie or whatever.

She was also democratic in her approach to our good health, and she chose to do what other mothers did as far as her conscience allowed. I remember an outbreak of scabies (itch) at school, and sure enough, we went home with red itching patches between our fingers. "It's not a disgrace to get the itch," Mother said, "but it is to keep it."

The generally accepted way to get rid of the itch was a ritualistic ordeal forced on all the kids in town—those with respectable mothers, that is. Every night we got a bath in hot water using homemade lye soap. Mother never made lye soap, but there was one woman in town who cleaned up (no pun intended) every year by selling lye soap when the itch struck the schoolhouse.

After the hot bath we were smeared with an ointment that had been stirred up in the kitchen. It consisted of lard, turpentine or kerosene, and powdered sulfur.

We then put on clean union suits and went to bed between clean sheets. Mother didn't do her own laundry, but in an emergency like that she boiled the sheets and union suits after each use in lots of water, stirring in some of the same lye soap she bought for our baths.

Needless to say, we didn't keep the itch very long. It was a blessing that Mother never got the idea that scabies was an internal poison that had to be cleaned out of our systems.

Even though she was astute in separating sham from reality, she did make a glaring mistake once. When my sister and I were in first grade, I outspelled everyone in the room and consequently was chosen to represent the class in the County Scholastic Meet. It was a big deal because I would get to ride the train 35 miles to the county seat.

I told my mother the morning we were to leave that I didn't feel so good. She felt my forehead and looked at my tongue and said it

The generally accepted way to get rid of the itch was a ritualistic ordeal forced on all the kids in town—those with respectable mothers, that is.

was probably a touch of tonsillitis. The trip was a big deal for Mother, too.

I made the trip with my teacher sitting on one side and my mother on the other, assuring each other that it was "probably a touch of tonsillitis." I received the gold medal for first prize—and exposed the whole county to mumps. But that was alright, because everyone should get the childhood diseases over with as early as possible—especially mumps.

Although my father agreed with my mother "in spirit and in truth," there were times when he tended to lose patience with some of her shenanigans in defense of healthy living.

My mother announced at the breakfast table one morning that she was going to buy some asafetida to have us wear around our necks.

"No!" he said, furious. "You are not going to bring that stinking stuff into this house!"

"But all the other mothers are getting it for their children," she replied evenly. (I doubt she even blushed when she pulled that old line.)

"Let them," Dad replied, fire in his eyes. "If the rest of the kids are wearing it, ours won't have to."

For the benefit of those who are fortunate enough never to have been initiated, let me explain that asafetida was a gummy substance which was sewn into a small cloth bag and worn around the neck on a string. It was supposed to ward off contagious diseases. Of course, what it really warded off was everyone within smelling distance. Its efficacy was roughly comparable to the biblical warning cry, "Unclean! Leper!"

However, after the first lump of it appeared in the classroom, everyone smelled alike and we never noticed the difference. One lump per classroom would do it.

An old medical book describes asafetida as a malodorous gum resin scraped from the roots of a plant grown in Persia (roughly, modern Afghanistan). Actually, it surpassed "malodorous" by a country mile. It smelled more like rotten onions and rotten garlic mixed together with rotten eggs.

Thanks to our father, we escaped asafetida, and its use faded elsewhere shortly thereafter. If asafetida were placed on one of those graphs we see occasionally in scientific magazines, it would fall somewhere after leeches and bloodletting and just before smallpox vaccinations.

My favorite druggist tells me that he still sells it, but in a liquid form. Some people buy it to use in making fish bait and others put it on poultices for chest colds. Well, nobody could deny that it opens the sinuses.

Mother, with Dad's assurance—if not his completely enthusiastic assistance—got us through school and married off. We never lost the benefits of the strong foundation she contributed on behalf of our staying well and enjoying robust good health.

While some of our peers might have had more tender-hearted parents, ours pointed with pride to the "perfect attendance" certificates awarded to us at the end of nearly every school term. It became a family joke that if we intended to get sick, we had best do it on a weekend so we wouldn't miss school. But we had no wish to spend our free weekends in boredom, lying in a dark bedroom, or "getting our systems cleaned out."

My siblings and I have spent a combined total of 99 years on this planet. Among the three of us we have experienced only five hospitalizations, and four of those were visits to the maternity ward. Our brother had surgery to remove scar tissue from a duodenal ulcer which

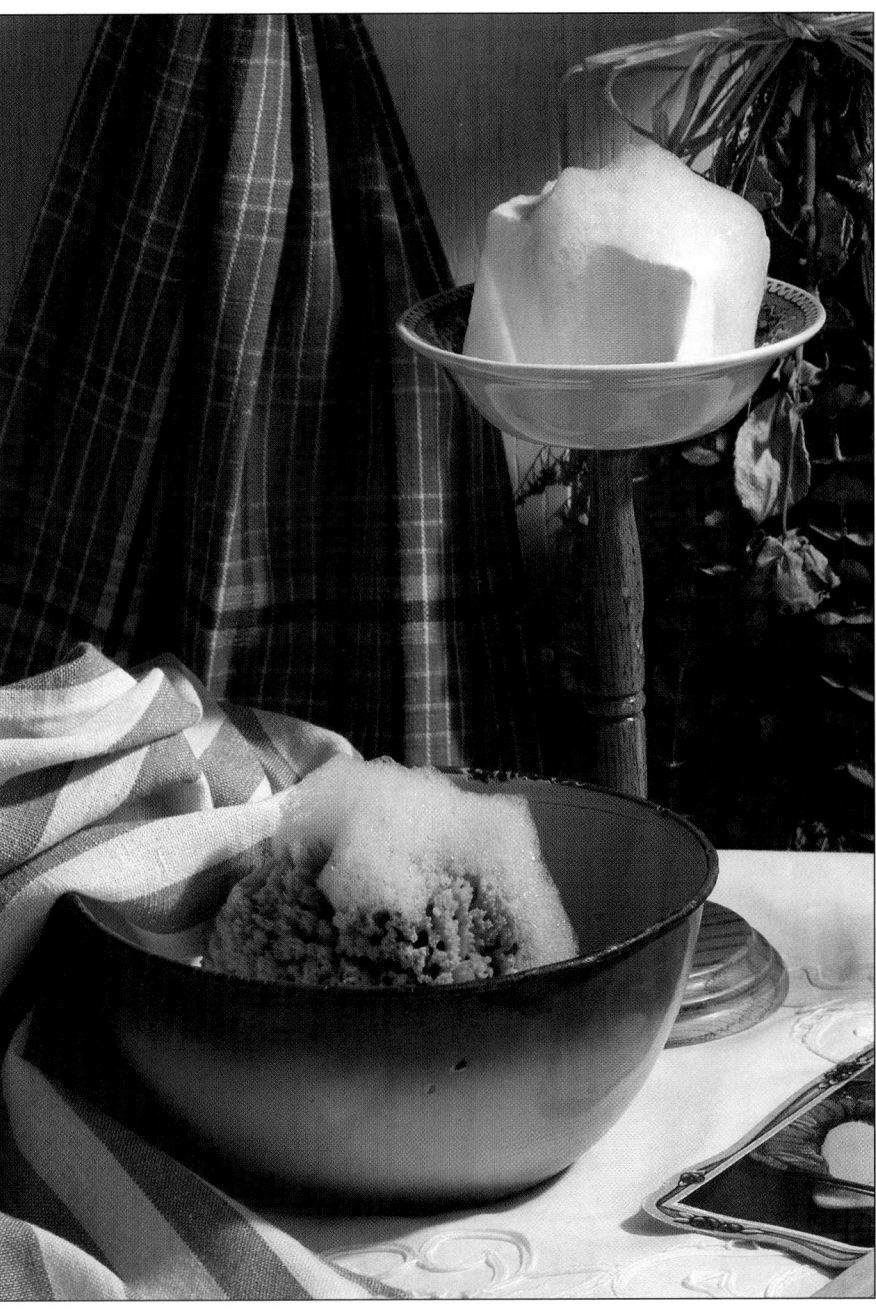

had healed and stopped up his works.

Mother died at age 79. During the last 10 years of her life, she suffered terribly from rheumatoid arthritis, but with the help of daily medication she stayed on her feet and cared for herself.

I teased her occasionally about being as cranky as a sore-tailed cat and threatened to withhold her dessert, but I would have done anything to ease her pain—anything. In my house, she could have had apple pie at midnight, and she knew it. ◆

Herbing

By Danny C. Blevins

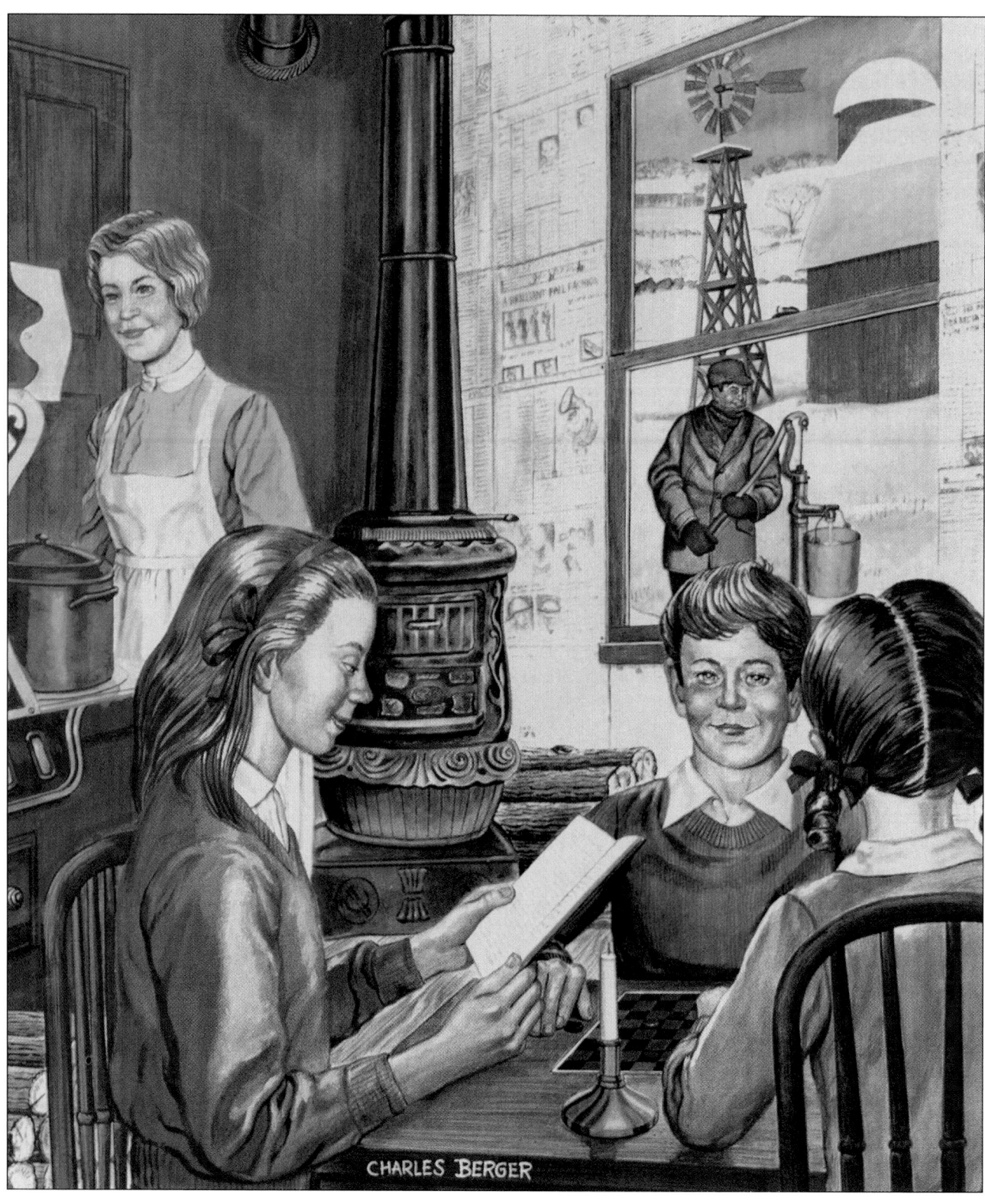

CHARLES BERGER

We called it "herbing," but I guess others in another part of the world referred to it by some other name. In the Tennessee mountains of my youth, the leaves, bark, roots and herbs of the plants and trees played an important part in our lives. They provided us with remedies for our coughs, soothed our sore throats, and comforted our bellyaches. But more importantly for my family, they provided us with a way to make a living during a time when money was more than tight— it was almost nonexistent.

One of my earliest childhood memories is of following my mother and father to the mountains to collect witch-hazel leaves, peel the bark of cherry trees, or collect log moss to sell to the local herb dealer. With our burlap sacks slung confidently over our shoulders, we would scour the mountain ridges and glens until our sacks were filled, we were too tired to continue, or there was nothing left to collect.

In the early spring, just as winter was loosening her death grip on the land, we would collect or "pull" log moss. Pieces as small as a man's hand and as big as a '55 Chevy were collected together and hung on fence railings to dry. Then it was neatly folded and pressed into 3-foot bales which we tied together with baling string and sold. In those days one man could make a good living by gathering moss, and many did.

When summer arrived, moss was forgotten because it was hard to spot in the lush, green mountains. But other herbs filled the needs of my family. We peeled the outer bark from the witch-hazel tree, then dried it and sold it, along with cherry bark and the bark from the roots of sassafras trees. We also dug mayapple roots and ginger plants to clean, dry and sell, but every dollar earned digging these roots was earned indeed.

The most important part of the summer gathering of herbs was collecting witch-hazel and sassafras leaves. In June and July, we collected these by the sackful, then dried them and sold them for 30, 40 or even 50 cents per pound. My goal during those hot summer months was to collect enough witch-hazel leaves to buy my back-to-school clothes. Even today, I remember how proud I felt the first summer I was able to buy them without taking money from my mother and father.

As the trees changed to dark green and then to hues of red, yellow and brown, we knew it was fall and time for one of my favorite pastimes, hunting ginseng. To us and many others, ginseng was an almost mystical plant which promised a small fortune for its root and was most enjoyable to dig. To a 10-year-old boy, no plant of the mountains could match its beauty as it hovered in the foliage, glistening with dew and drooping from the cherry-red berries which hung in the center of the plant. To this day I can still see the first plant I ever found by myself, sparkling in the shady light of the woods, and I can almost feel the pounding of my heart as I bent to dig its root. At $80 per dried pound, ginseng provided more than one meal for our table and put more than one pair of shoes on my feet.

During the long winter, snow, cold and frozen ground kept us in the house. I can remember looking through frosted windows at the snow-crusted mountains and wishing I could go into them to find what they had to offer. As the cold winter days blew past, we thought about our adventures in the mountains and told tales about the moss we had pulled and the ginseng root that was as big as a man's hand and about the heat and thirst of the summer. But through all the stories, we knew we enjoyed the life and would live no other way.

I am glad that I grew up in the mountains and was taught to "herb" for my clothes, food and other necessities of life. Herbing instilled in me a love for the mountains and creatures which inhabit them that has never left me. I still live in those mountains, and sometimes, just for fun and old times' sake, I go into the mountains again to dig ginseng or pull moss. This time I am not there for the money but for the enjoyment and for the memories.

During those days of long ago, herbing taught me the value of a dollar and helped us provide for our needs while giving us an appreciation of the wilderness and a storehouse of memories and stories which have lasted a lifetime. I am sure the well of my remembrances of those days will never run dry. ◆

When Mother's Sick

When Mother's sick, the house is all
So strangely hushed in room and hall,
But Mother never will admit
She's suffering a single bit.
She won't let people do a thing;
There's nothing anyone can bring.
She just lies there and tries to fix
Herself by cunning little tricks,
And as for a doctor, why the word
She scorns as being most absurd,
And when he comes, he's apt to say,
"You should have had me long before.
It's bed, you see, a week or more."

When Father's Sick

When Father's sick, I tell you now,
You ought to hear the dreadful row,
The talk of dying and the groans,
The orders in convulsive tones,
The hasty runners to and fro,
To rearrange the pillows so,
To fix hot-water bags and sage,
Mustard plasters, lemonade,
Appeals to get the doctor quick,
"For can't you see, I'm awful sick."
And when he comes, he just says, "Hum,
"Unless I'm needed, I shan't come.
"I think he'll do all right."
And Father's up, perhaps by night.

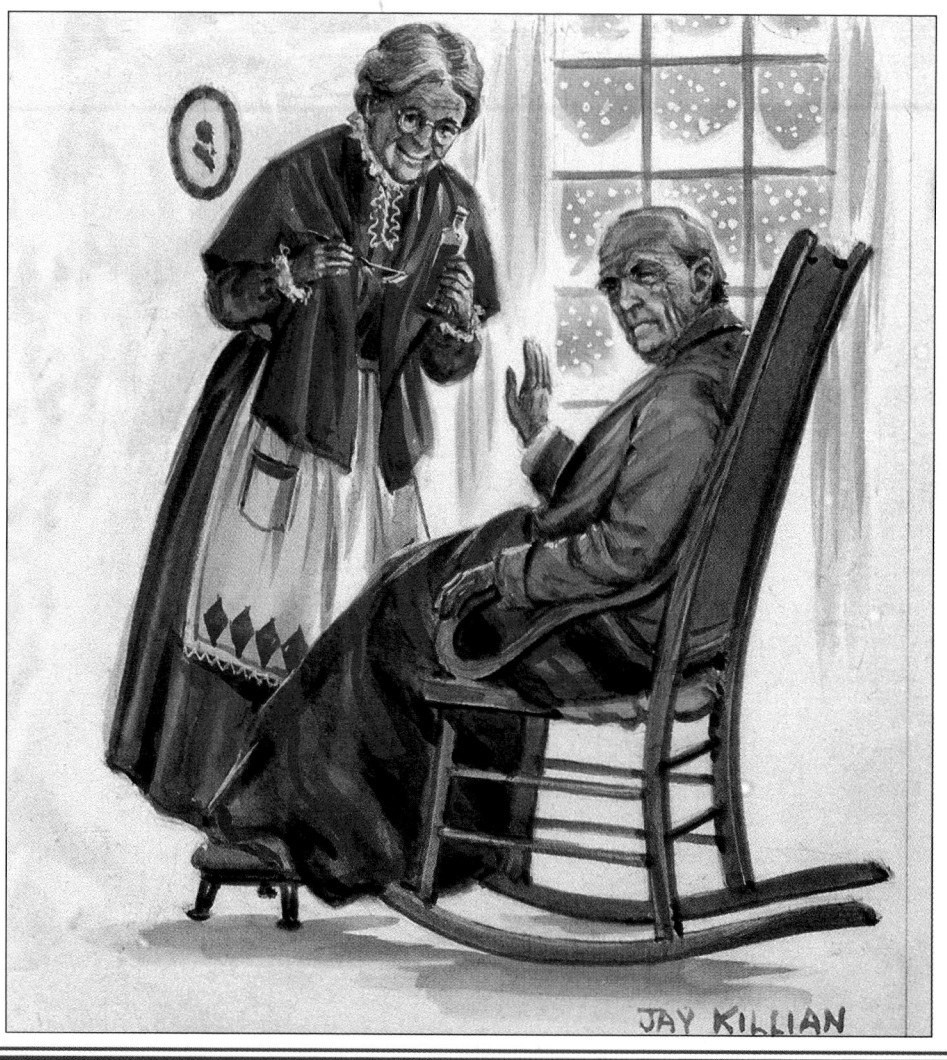

JAY KILLIAN

Chapter 3

TONICS AND OTHER CURES

Remember when Lydia Pinkham's product for women promised "a baby in every bottle"? How many youngsters back in the Good Old Days secreted away a bottle of Lydia's tonic, figuring at last they had found out where babies came from? Genies came out of bottles, why not babies?

Uncle Bob found me with a bottle of it, looking for a little brother. Without getting into the birds and the bees, he gently explained that "a baby in every bottle" was a slogan, not a promise.

The tonics of yesterday promised to cure everything from baldness to digestive problems, from rashes to respiratory ailments. Some had at least scientific basis. Some were harmless. Some were enough to make the bravest kid run for cover. These stories will remind you of the days when your mother asserted, "Of course it tastes awful, it's medicine!"

—Ken Tate

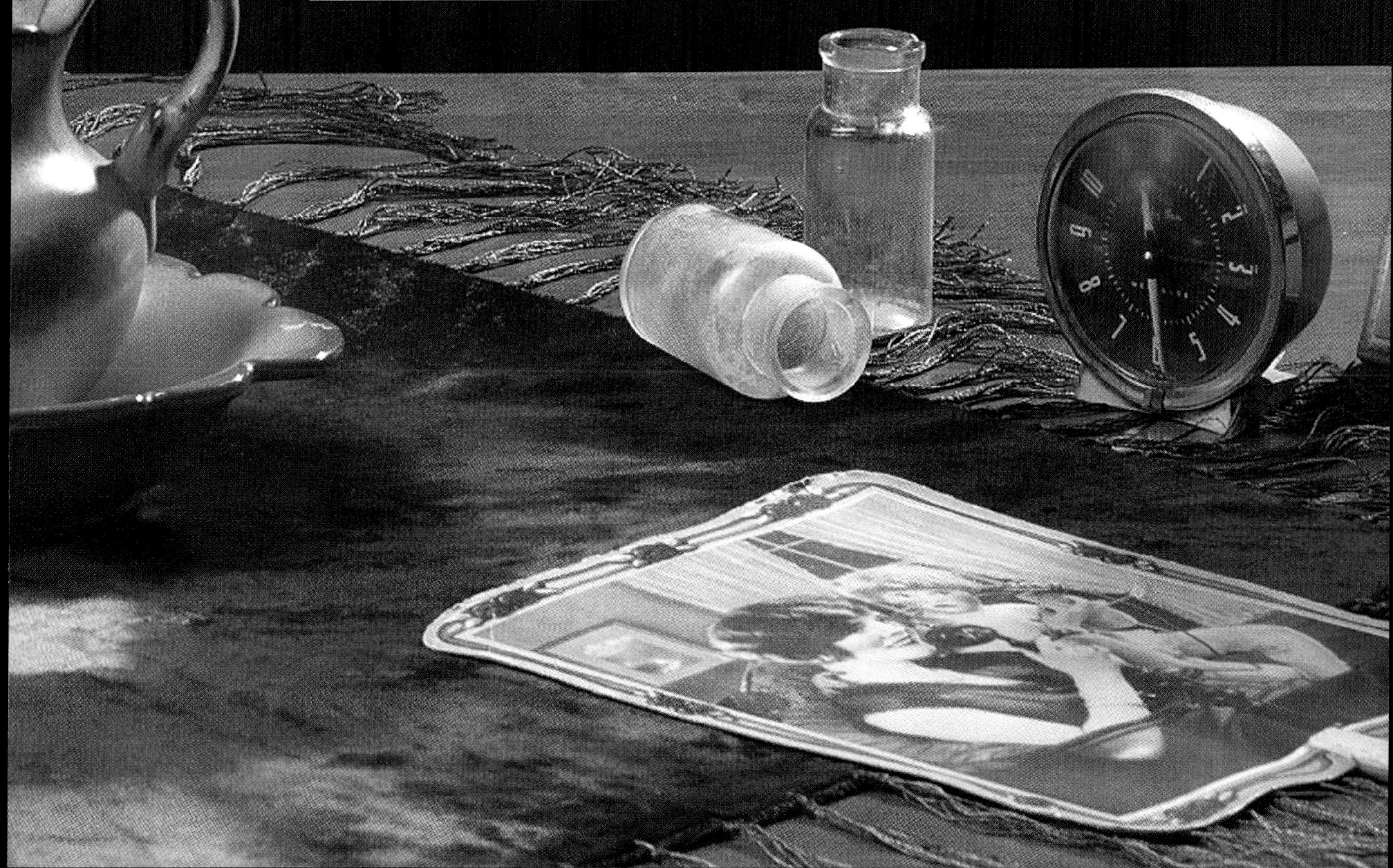

That Winter Scalp Treatment

By Carol Ann Jensen

One cold, wintry December day we moved from a little one-room house on Grandpa's farm into a bigger house with possibilities on a newly purchased farm in a little Idaho town.
Working from early morning until late at night left us exhausted and out of touch with our neighbors—either from our old home west of Gooding or our new neighbors to the east.

It was 1941 and our area was sparsely settled, so we had neither electricity nor telephone when we moved in. But Daddy made arrangements with the power company to hook up electricity within the coming week.

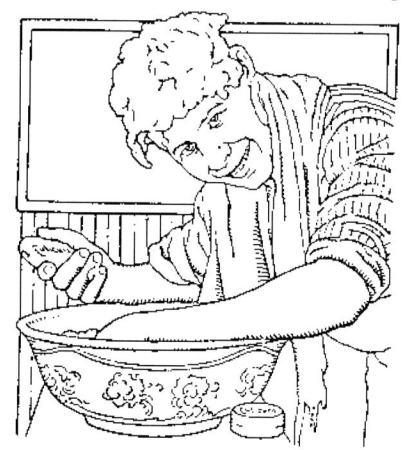

We wanted and needed electricity; after all, we had been accustomed to using it in our old home. However, Daddy had a very special reason for wanting the electricity. He had received an electric scalp massager for Christmas the previous year, and how he did love it! "I need electricity to run my scalp vibrator," Daddy said. "I don't want to get bald this early in life, so I must massage my scalp." His head of shiny red hair was his pride and joy.

So Dad had the house wired with plugs, including an extra one in the bathroom just for his scalp vibrator.

He hung the new pink chandeliers for the family to enjoy. Mother wiped all the fingerprints from the switches so they would be clean and shiny for the maiden flip-on. She even shined up Daddy's vibrator plug-in.

"Now don't one of you touch these switches," she cautioned in a voice that left no room for doubt or disagreement.

The next day a new neighbor stopped by to bring us good tidings, greetings from the neighborhood, and the not-so-good news about the state of world affairs. "Yesterday, December 7," he said, "Japan bombed Pearl Harbor! We now are at war!"

Later that day we had another visitor, with more bad news. "Due to the war, we'll be unable to hook up your power this week," he said. "We don't even know when we can hook it up; possibly not until after the war."

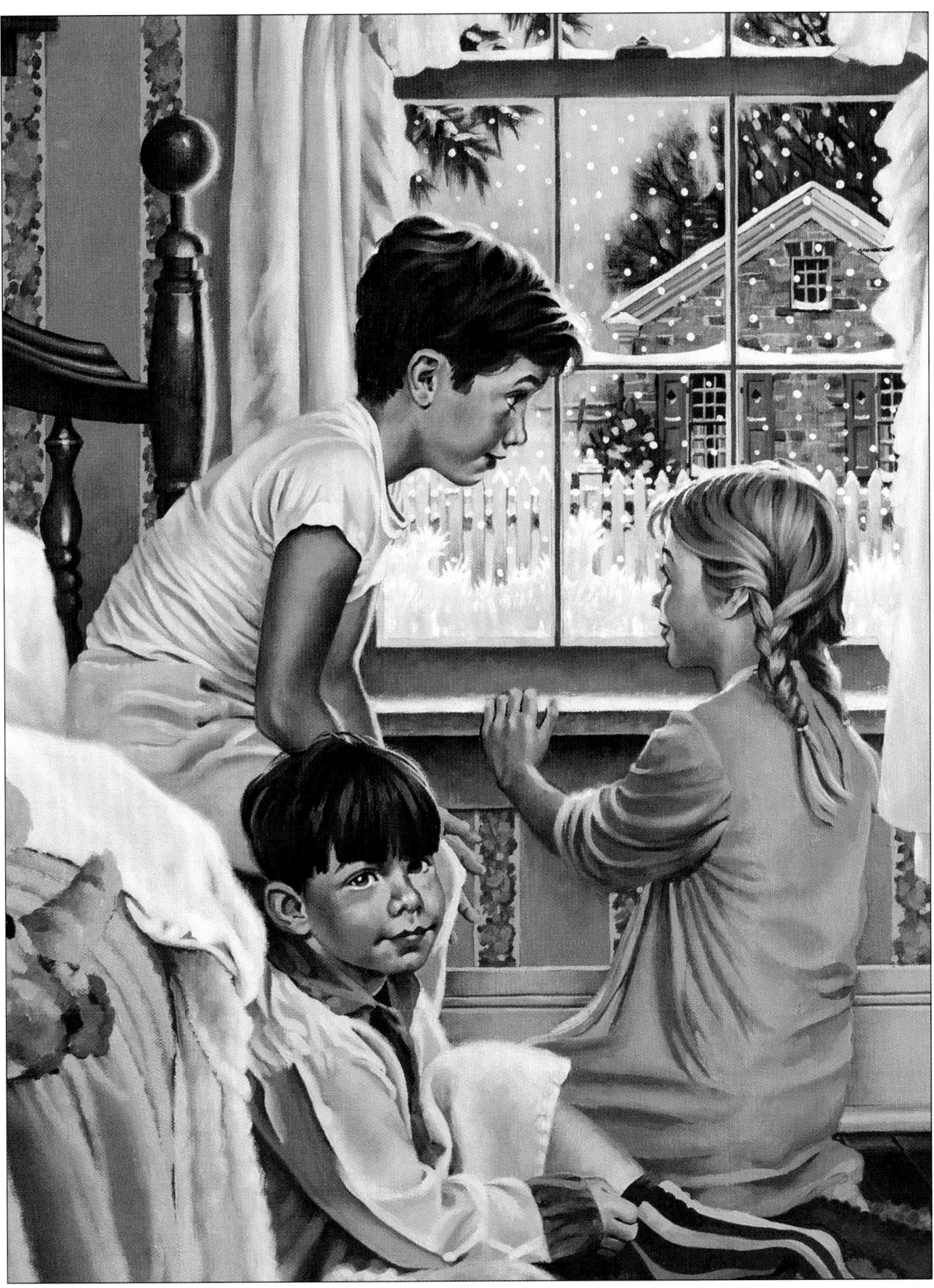

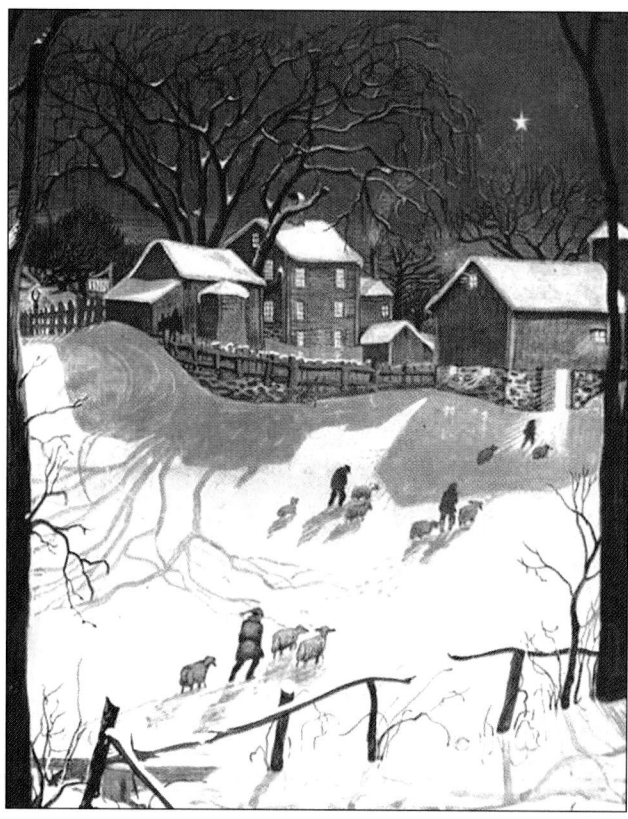

Mama groaned.

Daddy appealed to the power officials and pleaded with them as only he could do. He made every possible effort to get them to carry the power from the main line to our house only a few yards away.

But it was all to no avail. Daddy couldn't use his scalp vibrator. Now he would have to give himself a scalp treatment with his big hands and long fingers.

The pink chandeliers hung dark from the high ceiling in the front room. For several years they watched as we ate, slept, remodeled, practiced piano and gave parties, all by the light of old kerosene pump-up lanterns—the kind with the silk mantles that looked like perfect stockings for my dollies, if ever I could figure a way to get a pair into my own hot little hands.

Carrying the faithful old lantern was a ritual—a part of nearly every activity. We carried it from room to room in the house, hooking it above the sink or over the piano. We carried it from the house to the barn to finish late chores. If members of the family were busy in different rooms, it meant either lighting another lamp or working in the dark. Often,

rather than light an extra lamp, any task which might be completed without a light was at least tried with the touch-and-grope method.

"Put thumb firmly over air hole in attached pump," read the instructions. "Pump until pressure feels adequate. Turn on the jet and immediately touch lighted match to mantles." It always broke me up to watch Daddy touch a match to the "dolly socks."

"I wish I could plug in my vibrator," Daddy said. "I need a scalp treatment. Guess a manual massage is better than none, though," and he worked down through the thick red hair to wiggle his scalp. He finished with a dab of hair oil.

One Saturday night we had all been invited to a party at a house in town. Town homes had electricity, and it was always such fun to flick the light switches off and on, off and on—when Mom wasn't looking.

We were all ready to go, except Daddy. "Hurry, Daddy, let's go," we chided from the living room. All dressed and polished, we were trying very hard to sit still as commanded by Mother so we couldn't get "mussed."

Mother was in the bedroom getting a kerchief for Daddy. This was one of those tasks performed by touch-and-grope. Only one lantern was lit, and no one wanted to take the time to light another. Daddy offered, but we told him we didn't need it.

"Never mind lighting one for me, dear," Mama assured him. "I can put my hands right on those kerchiefs. I just ironed and put them away today." As organized and tidy as Mama was, I knew she could lay a hand on anything in the house with both eyes shut. So they left the lantern in the front room for us kids so we wouldn't fidget.

The light threw shadows which danced and flickered on the walls. We giggled and made pictures in the shadows.

While Mama was after the kerchief, Daddy decided to put on a little more hair oil and give his scalp a quick massage. "I'll tell you, Mama," he declared, "this oil isn't as good as it used to be. I'd better put just another touch on my hair. What do you think?"

"Whatever you think, Daddy," Mama replied sweetly. She knew how proud Daddy was of his wavy red hair. "There may be a few strands misbehaving."

Daddy started for the big kitchen where the medicine chest was bolted high on the wall. It was full of remedies—a bottle of cough medicine, a tube of lipstick, a little face powder and some lotions and creams for Mama, as well as Daddy's shaving mug and razor, a bottle of hair oil and some after-shave lotion.

On his way from the bedroom to the kitchen, Daddy passed through the front room where we were sitting, impatient to get going and growing more restless with every minute. He reached for the lamp.

"No, no!" we shouted. "Don't take our light! We're using it right now!"

Being naturally good-humored, Daddy was in an extra-lenient mood and set the lamp back on the table. "OK, you kids," he chortled, "but it's only because you're being good kids that I will leave it here. Just wait a few more minutes while I have a scalp treatment and a dab of oil. Then I'll be ready to go."

He walked into the kitchen.

There was a little bump as Daddy passed the shiny new Monarch range. It was all-white—nice enough, but still inconvenient compared to the electric one we had anticipated.

Shortly we heard another little bump. "Daddy isn't as familiar with the kitchen as Mama is," I said.

"Should we take him the light?" we whispered to one another. But we voted against it; we were having such fun making shadow pictures.

Mama had found the kerchief without a light and was coming into the front room. We heard Daddy open the medicine chest in the kitchen, take out a bottle, then noisily unscrew the lid. Then we heard a yell.

"Woman!" bellowed Daddy. (He only called Mama that in that tone of voice when he was very upset.)

Of course, we all rushed into the kitchen, light in hand, dreading what had happened to Daddy.

What we saw shocked us.

Daddy was standing there with an indescribable expression on his face, holding a bottle in his hand. It was the same size and shape as the bottle his hair oil came in.

But it wasn't hair oil. It was cough syrup. The sticky, sweet-smelling syrup was on Daddy's hands and in his hair. It literally covered his head.

We didn't dare laugh or cry or hardly even breathe. No one moved for what seemed like an eternity.

"Please, Daddy, don't make us stay home and miss the party!" Then, hoping against hope and the inevitable, we all cried.

Daddy had a very special reason for wanting the electricity. He had received an electric scalp massager for Christmas the previous year, and how he did love it!

Mama soothed. "Now Daddy, it will only take a minute to fix up your messy head." She began bustling around, but all the heated water from the water jacket on the range had been used for our baths earlier. We had let the fire go out, and there was no more hot water in the tank.

How will we ever wash sticky cough syrup out of Daddy's hair with a dab of lukewarm water? I wondered.

But Mama worked wonders with washcloths. She did the best she could, then assured Daddy that his hair was clean, shiny and even fresh-smelling.

"I still feel sweet and sticky," Daddy moaned.

"Now, now," Mama clucked. "Let's just put a dab of hair oil on to tame down a few of these mischievous strands of hair, and then we'll be off to the party."

Daddy groaned but agreed to take us.

It seems to me that I remember that Daddy's hair was extra-shiny and glossy for a few days after that episode. Maybe that cough-syrup scalp treatment was just what Daddy needed! At any rate, it was many years before Daddy did go bald.

"After that night," he remembered with a laugh, "my hair just 'stuck around.'" ◆

Steam Bath

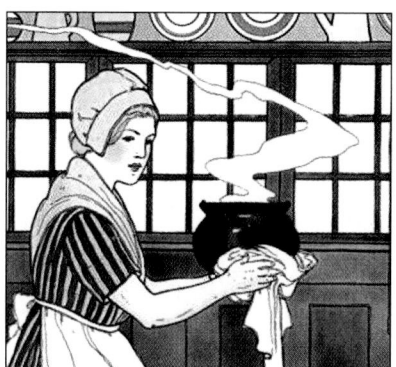

By Lois Greene Stone

Want to comfort a cold? I recently read in a magazine article that steaming the face can ease mild congestion from a cold especially when fragrant oils are added to the water. I smiled as I scanned this "new" idea.

Even before decongestants and antibiotics, my mother treated colds, sinus infections and any other head ailment the same way. So it's come full circle.

I can still visualize this incident from the 1940s:

"Whatever are you doing?" My mother passed by the bathroom, shook her head and smiled. "You're supposed to be inhaling vapors to get rid of your sinus congestion. Inhale. Stop singing." She pretended to be giving a stern order, but it was playful.

"Chickory chick, cha la, cha la," I chanted as I wiggled the towel that formed a tent over my head. "Cha la, cha la." Then I sang, "What shall I do with my mother, mommy, ma?" I giggled at the rhyming.

My mother tapped my small behind. "Steam!"

The porcelain basin was filled to the drain-out hole. Chamomile leaves in the hot water gave the concoction a characteristic odor. I didn't think it was fragrant, but rather smelly. I'd drunk tea with chamomile leaves and detangled my hair with a mixture of chamomile and water—and now I had to inhale its moist fumes.

Appearing in the doorway again, my mother commanded, *"Now. Before the water gets cold."*

"OK, OK," I whined. "Yuk!" I bent over the sink, replacing the terry-towel tent over my head, and inhaled. I wanted to keep my eyes closed so I wouldn't have to stare at the small cracks in the sink, the stains that remained even after cleaners, the film that formed on the water's surface. But if I pressed my eyelids together too long, I felt dizzy, then imagined my head plopping into porcelain and drowning in misty droplets.

"You sure look weird." My older sister, Carole, came up behind me. "I'm lucky I never get sinus infections."

"You sure look weird," my older sister Carole said. "I'm lucky I never get sinus infections."

I pulled myself straight and let the towel drop onto my shoulders. "I don't have 'hay fever, a-choo,' stupid."

Looking at my red, puffy face, Carole laughed and walked away.

Uncertain about what she was laughing at, I felt angry. I released the lever and watched the water drain away. I couldn't see my reflection in the steamy mirror, so I wiped a small section clear with my towel. My silky hair was moist and matted. My cheeks were slightly swollen. "I'd rather be congested," I told my image.

"I'd rather not be up all night with you," my mother responded.

"Can't I even have a conversation with myself without being overheard!" I rolled up the towel and forced it down the metal laundry chute, then stuck my head near to watch it flop into a wicker basket a floor below.

My mother laughed. "Come help me fix dinner. It's better than a mustard plaster when you get chest colds, isn't it?"

"Are you kidding? Breathing smelly vapors, bent over a sink. And it has been 'Laugh at Lois Day' and now you want my help?" Then, with a dramatic gesture, I added, "*Dah*-ling, I am too sick with sinus trouble to peel potatoes. Ask your healthy older daughter. It isn't hay fever season."

My mother continued to chuckle, then called, "Carole?"

Now, five decades later, for those who don't want to take medication for congestion, inhaling steam from a mixture of hot water and scented oil is again being promoted as an option. And chamomile tea is back. I wonder if mustard plasters will …

Nah. ◆

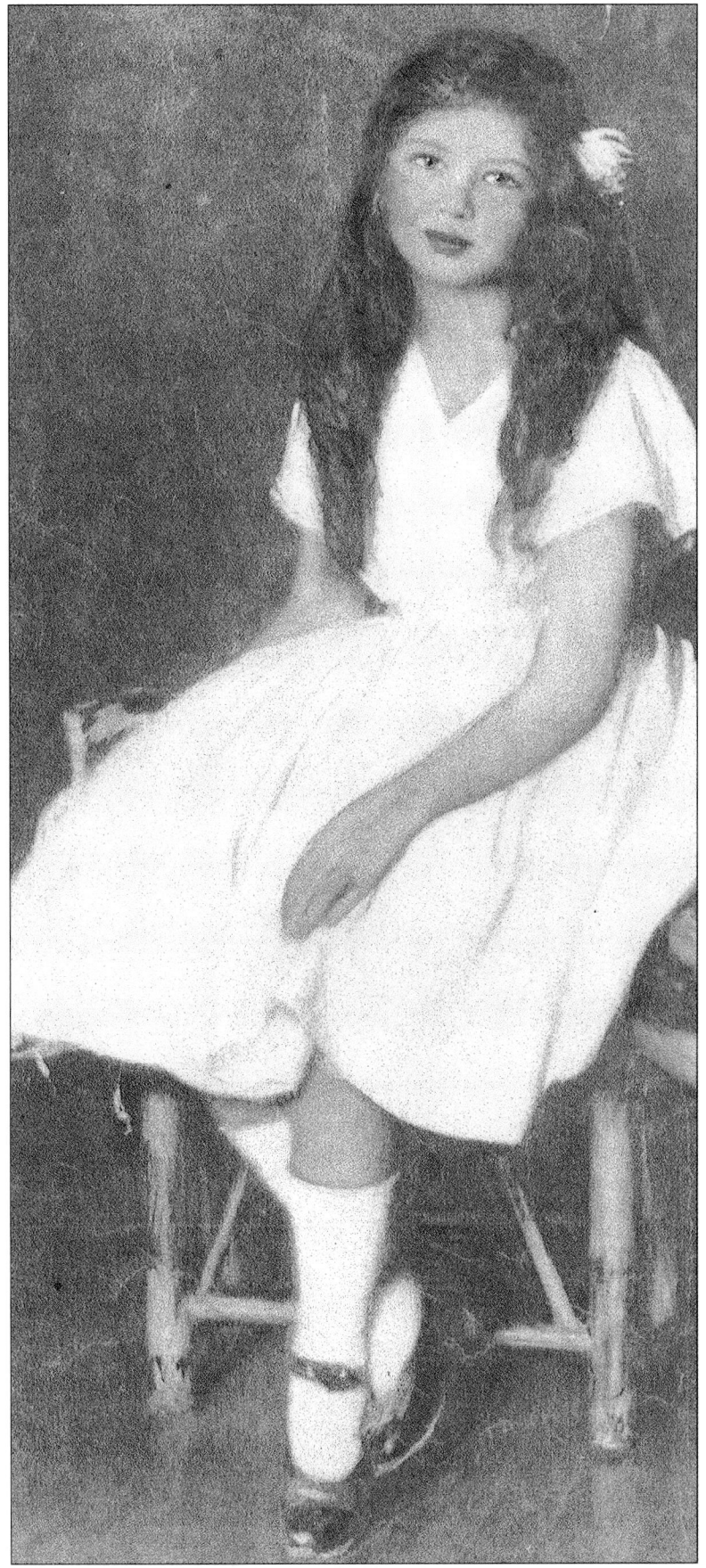

How to Keep Well In 1909

By Alice Harnish

Onions are almost the best nervine known. No medicine is so useful in cases of nervous prostration, and there is nothing else that will so quickly relieve and tone up a worn-out system. Onions are useful in all cases of coughs, colds and influenza, in consumption, insomnia, hydrophobia and scurvy. Eaten every other day they very soon have a clearing and whitening effect on the complexion."

So states Joseph P. Bushnell in *What To Do And How To Do It*, a home manual compiled by him "after years of extensive research" and published in 1909. The book, originally my grandmother's, covers the home, health and culinary art, care of the sick, the farm and its activities and business law. One finds an interesting blend of old-fashioned and modern ideas.

Vegetables as medicine seems a quaint notion to us now, but the book's long list includes carrots for asthma, tomatoes and pie plants as "aperients" (his word for laxative), olives for stimulating blood circulation, celery as a sedative and blackberries for diarrhea (still recommended).

In his manual, Mr. Bushnell claimed that 90 percent of all illness is due to ignorance, carelessness and intemperance.

"Good health and longevity require a healthy condition of the stomach, a healthy nervous system and muscular action, and a proper system of drainage. To maintain these conditions nature has provided abundantly pure air, pure water, sunlight and good food. We must also assure cleanliness, temperance, exercise and rest."

He believed in the influence of the mind over the body. "Energy is primarily a thing of the mind and spirit. Many have the habit of not feeling well. Some are chronic complainers, dwelling continually upon their aches and pains until they become actually increased. Of course," he concedes, "a person's mental condition does often to a considerable extent depend upon the bodily condition."

Recommendations include: "Keep your thoughts away from morbid subjects; fix them upon the healthful, the joyous, the beautiful. The world is full of beauty, sunshine and happiness. Meet happy people.

Onions are useful in treating many illnesses. Eaten every other day they very soon have a clearing and whitening effect on the complexion.

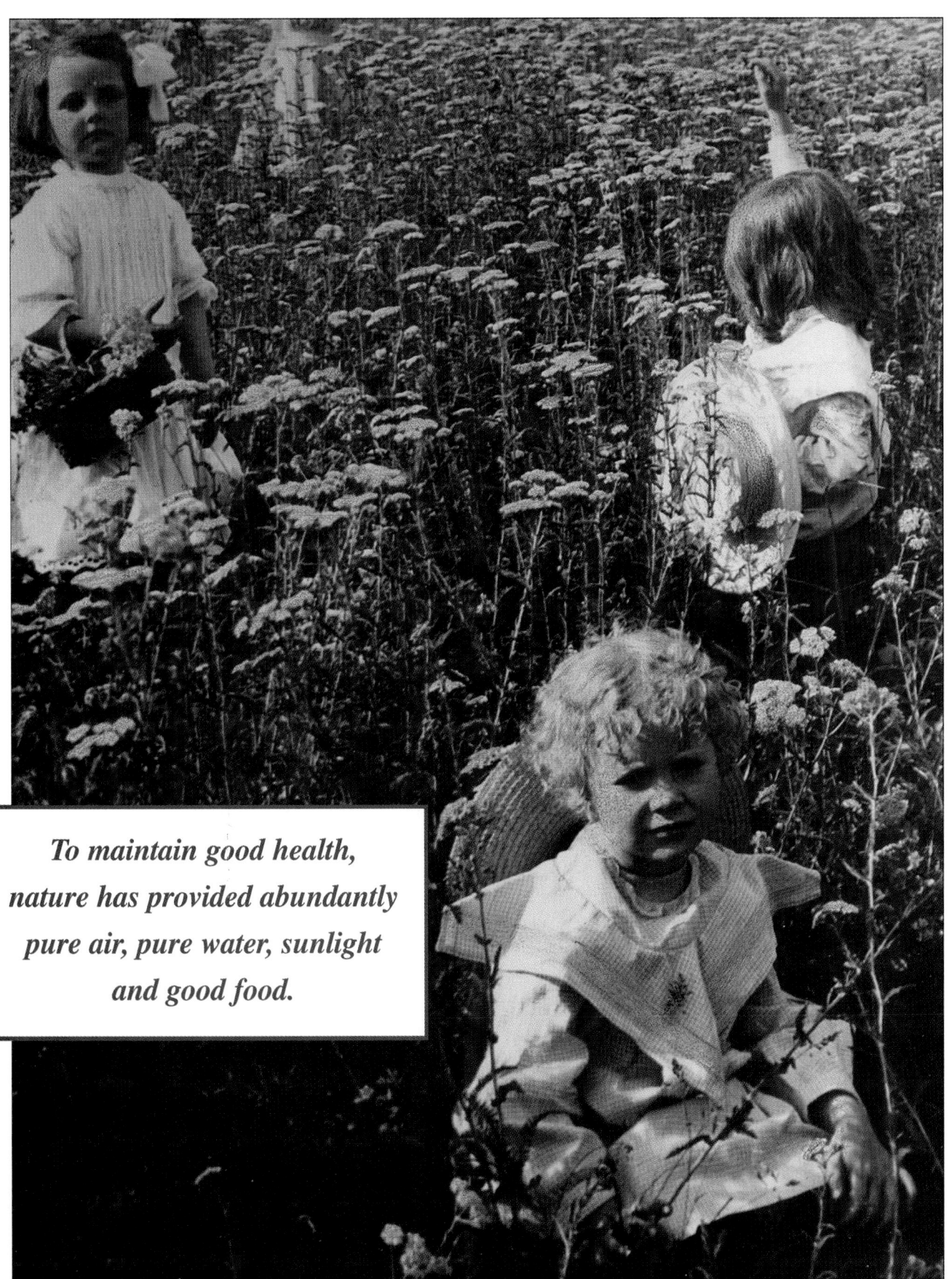

To maintain good health, nature has provided abundantly pure air, pure water, sunlight and good food.

Smile. Make yourself useful. Don't worry. Be courageous. What is grit and pluck but the everlasting insistence that things are bound to come out right some way?"

Breathe properly, he says. "We are a nation of lazy breathers. Fill the lungs, using the diaphragm muscle, not the muscles of the upper thorax. Keep chest elevated and abdomen drawn in; do not raise the shoulders or chest. Be outdoors as much as possible, get fresh air constantly into the house. And," he adds, "the air is always purer when it snows or rains." (Acid rain was unknown in 1909.)

Readers are told they must vary their diet, and avoid overeating, over-prepared foods and "piecing." They must eat raw fresh fruits and vegetables (as is advised today).

"Avoid foods excessively cooked or soaked in fat. The frying pan is the great American evil."

However, some other advice seems inconsistent. In a table of times required for cooking, we read: "Boil asparagus 20 to 30 minutes, young cabbage 45, carrots one hour, dandelions one and a half hours, spinach 30 minutes, string beans 2 hours."

For proper digestion and to avoid "costiveness" (his word for constipation), we are told to chew each mouthful 30 times, a process called "Fletcherizing" after its proponent, Dr. Horace Fletcher. A paragraph on "diet of old age" includes the dismaying news that it should usually be very similar to that of childhood—quite bland.

As for temperance: "Drinking and smoking must be avoided. Cigarettes are a rapid, powerful poison. To terminate the liquor habit, at least three apples eaten a day will gradually end the horrible craving," according to a physician quoted in the *Philadelphia Bulletin*. A correspondent in the *Waverley Magazine* stated that five or six glasses of buttermilk will help. (Incidentally, 2 quarts of good buttermilk a day will cure any case of nervous indigestion.)

Exercise abundantly, we are urged. Walking is very good. Also advocated are running, horseback riding (women should ride astride), bicycling, rowing, skating, swimming and games. Be outdoors as much as possible; always breathe fresh air. Exercise indoors too. The author gives some exercises just for women, not as strenuous as those for men. He wrote, "Gym classes these days are filling up rapidly."

"To secure refreshing sleep take nothing more exciting than chocolate or weakest tea before bedtime, never coffee, strong tea or wine. Sip hot milk, take a lukewarm sponge bath; don't go to bed with cold feet. Have windows open. Don't sleep in a draft. Go to bed to sleep, not to read, write or think."

However, if your problem should be sleepwalking, this is the advice given: "Place a tub half or quarter full of cold water in front of bed or couch. When the subject gets out of bed and puts feet in the water, he or she will awaken at once. Do this until cured, or tack pieces of oilcloth on the floor at the side of the bed. When stepped upon, the contact of the feet with the cold will cause the sleepwalker to awake."

Rest in the daytime is also necessary, said Mr. Bushnell. "Lie down, in the middle of the day preferably, even if only for 10 minutes or five. If you cannot lie down, lean back in a chair and close your eyes. Do not think over what has happened. Do not plan what is going to happen. Rest. Relax. See that there is no muscle tense anywhere. This practice will make you live longer. It will make you healthier while you do live. It will probably make people want you to live longer." ◆

Strange Medicine

By Louise Foster Pate

As we were growing up we were dosed with anything and everything. Most of it was foul-tasting. A spoonful of medicine was followed by a graham cracker, or it was taken with orange juice. We never questioned a dose of cocoa quinine, syrup of figs or senna tea.

Dad himself constantly imbibed one preparation after another. Alka Seltzer stood side-by-side with cough syrup on the shelf in the bathroom medicine cabinet.

My father was apt to act on the spur of the moment. One day I came upon him in the kitchen as he was pouring a spoonful of medicine from a strange bottle. "What are you taking?" I asked.

"Well, I don't know for sure, but I hope it will make me feel better," he said.

"You mean you are taking something you don't know about?" I asked. "Where did you get it?"

He explained that on Saturday he had taken his usual trip to town. He parked his car and went into the bank. When he returned to his car, there was a package in it and it contained, of all things, a bottle of patent medicine. Someone had mistaken Dad's Chevy for his own and had left the package there.

He didn't know whose it was and he was sorry about that. "I hate to see it go to waste," Dad said, "so I'm trying to see if it will do me some good."

I sought out Mother. She did not share Dad's faith in healing concoctions. I wondered what she thought about it.

"Oh well, don't worry. It's just a tonic, you know. He is like his mother who would take any cure she heard about."

When Dad was 21 he had typhoid fever. His family declared that ever since he had suffered from a weak stomach. Mother cut out greasy foods and served him whole-wheat bread, fresh fruits with honey and other recommended diet foods. He lived to be 88 years old. Was his long life a result of his diet—or patent medicine? ◆

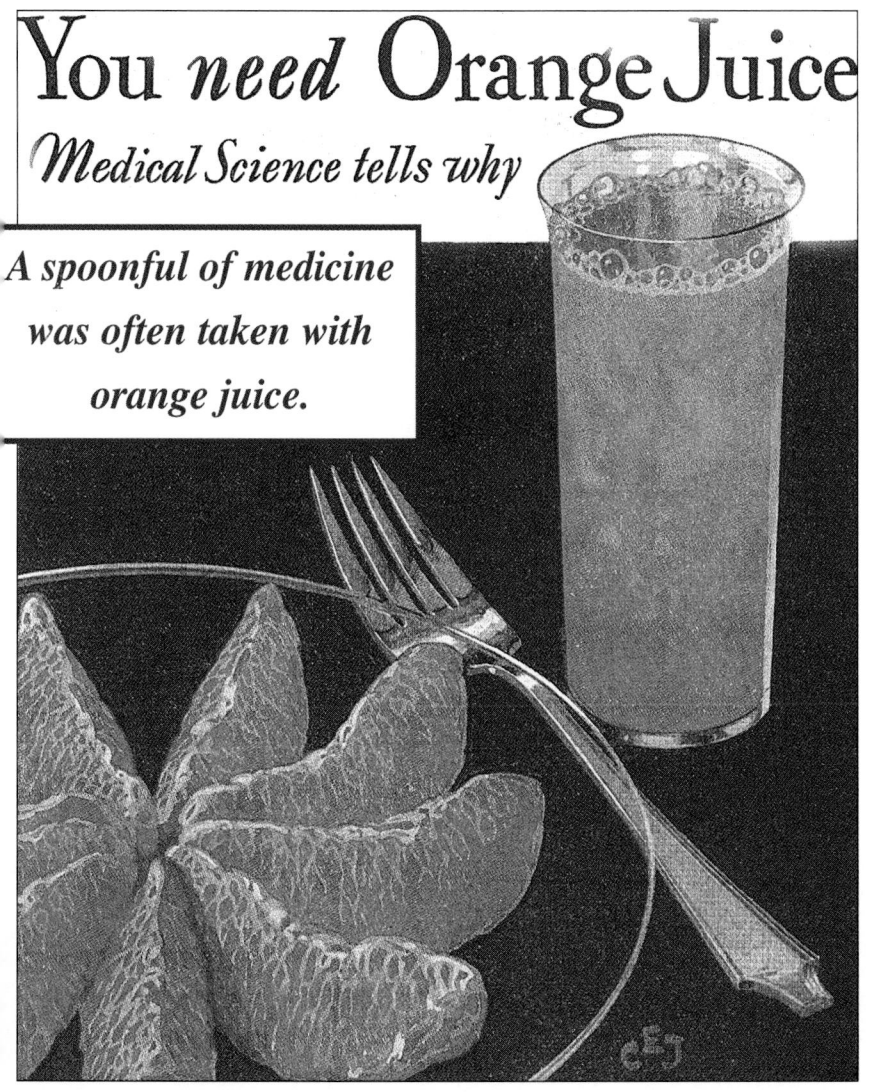

You *need* Orange Juice
Medical Science tells why

A spoonful of medicine was often taken with orange juice.

Dr. Tommy Scott's Last Real Medicine Show

By Janice Cole Gibson

Step right up and get your bottle of herbs, roots, barks and berries, gathered from all parts of the globe and blended into one mild yet effective tonic laxative! It's good for the entire family—the old folks, dads and all—and it's sold with a money-back guarantee!"

Doc Tom Scott's clear Southern voice called out the pitch for the old-time medicine show in the true barker's style. Wearing a bright striped shirt with garters on the sleeves, a vest, bow tie and top hat, he had worked the medicine show since 1936. His was the only medicine show still traveling the circuits of small towns across the United States and Canada when I saw it back in 1988.

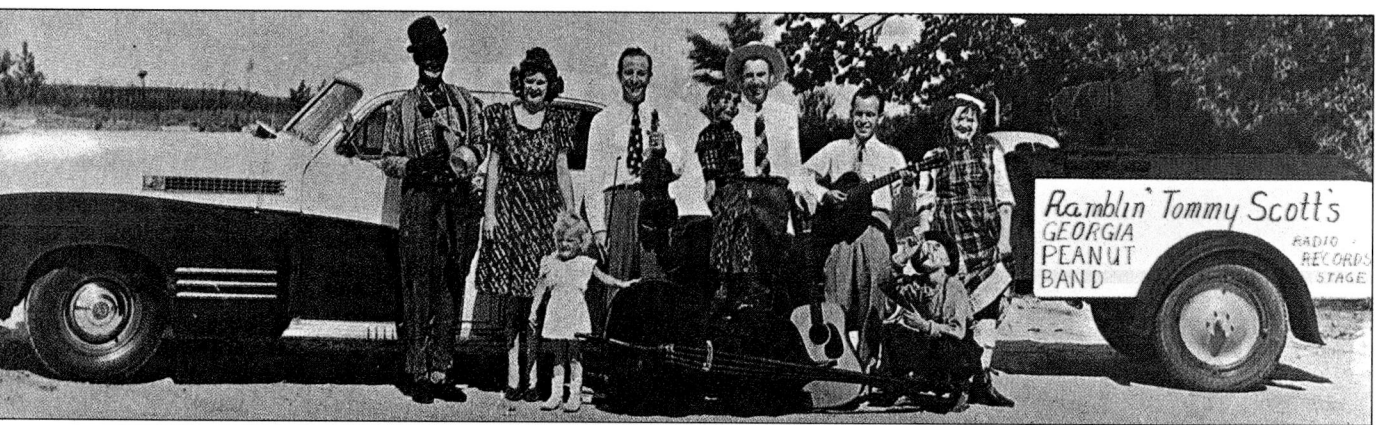

It all began for Tom Scott in 1936 when, as a lad of 16, he left his dad's corn and cotton fields in Toccoa, Ga., to join Doc Chamberlain's Medicine Show. Chamberlain came to Toccoa every year, so when news of that year's show spread, Tom picked up his guitar and headed for town. No one else showed up at the audition, so Tom was hired for $6 a week and told to meet the show in Eberton, Ga., in three weeks.

He walked and hitchhiked to Eberton in the warm fall weather, and found Doc Chamberlain repairing a platform for that night's performance.

"Hi, Mr. Chamberlain. I'm ready to go to work," Tom told him.

"What do you mean?" Chamberlain asked.

"I'm the boy you hired." Tom was beginning to get uneasy.

"Where?"

"In Toccoa," Tom replied.

Chamberlain laughed. He told Tom that everyone was always coming to him for jobs. When he hired them on the spot, he found that most of them ran off in a few days, leaving him short of help. So he told them to meet him down the road in a few weeks. Most of them never showed up, so Chamberlain had grown accustomed to forgetting about them.

"But I am here," Tom told him. "I have all my belongings in a paper bag and box." So Chamberlain told him he could sleep in the front of an old Dodge truck. Thus began Tom's long career.

Doc Tom Scott's clear Southern voice called out the pitch for the old-time medicine show in the true barker's style.

Tom picked and sang and became part of the medicine show. Chamberlain apparently took a real liking to him, for when he prepared to retire about a year and a half later, he gave Tom the formula for the medicine and asked him to carry on the tradition. And that's just what Tom did for more than 50 years.

The summer before he retired, Chamberlain and Tom pitched the show full time. In the fall, however, they would work only on weekends unless a trial or some other event brought more people into town. When Chamberlain decided to retire, he ran an ad in *Billboard* magazine, a publication for showmen, to find Tom a job to see him through until summer, when he could again pitch the show full time.

From the responses, Chamberlain picked a Raleigh, N.C., radio station. Chamberlain left for California and Tom never heard from him again.

At the Raleigh station Tom was hired by a dramatic show to add some of the picking and singing that was becoming so popular. In six months Scott was doing half the show due to the overwhelming response from the audience. Later the show went to an all-music format. During this time, Tom was still selling his

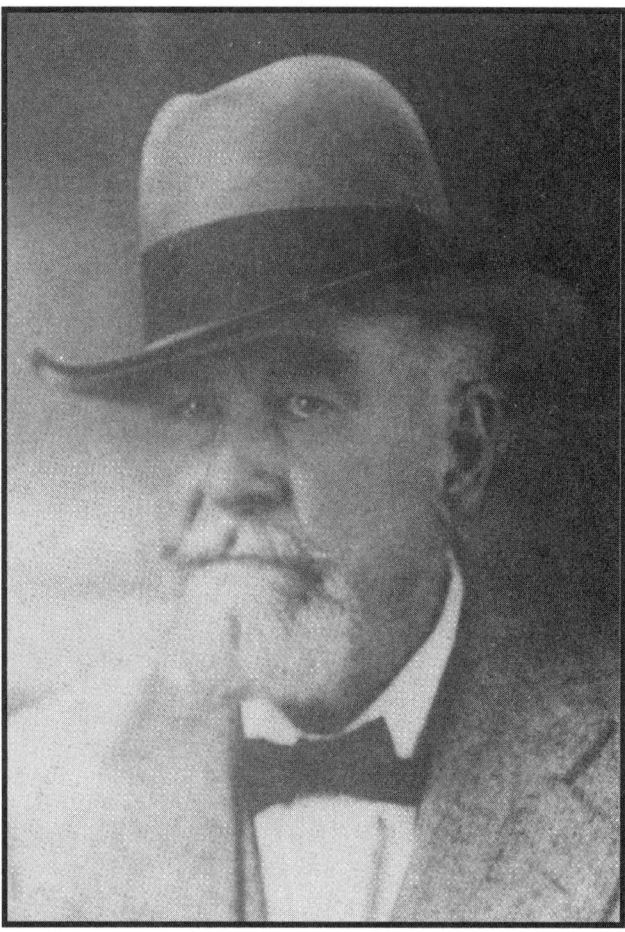

Doc M.F. Chamberlain, Dr. Tommy's predecessor

herbal medicine part time.

Shortly afterward, Tom joined Charlie Monroe when he and his brother, Bill, split up. When Charlie lost his sponsor, he and Tom began selling medicine over the air from Greensboro, N.C. They used Doc Chamberlain's formula, but they called it Mantoree.

Their program aired on more than a dozen radio stations from Georgia through the Carolinas and into Virginia. But Tom didn't receive the money they had agreed upon, so he left and took his formula with him.

Tom had actually received two recipes from Doc Chamberlain—one for Herb-O-Lac, an herbal laxative, and another for Snake Oil, a liniment for external application. Chamberlain had concocted both formulas in the 1800s with the help of a Cherokee Indian. Both are made with natural ingredients.

Doc Scott vouched for the medicine—it was indeed formulated to do what it is proclaimed to

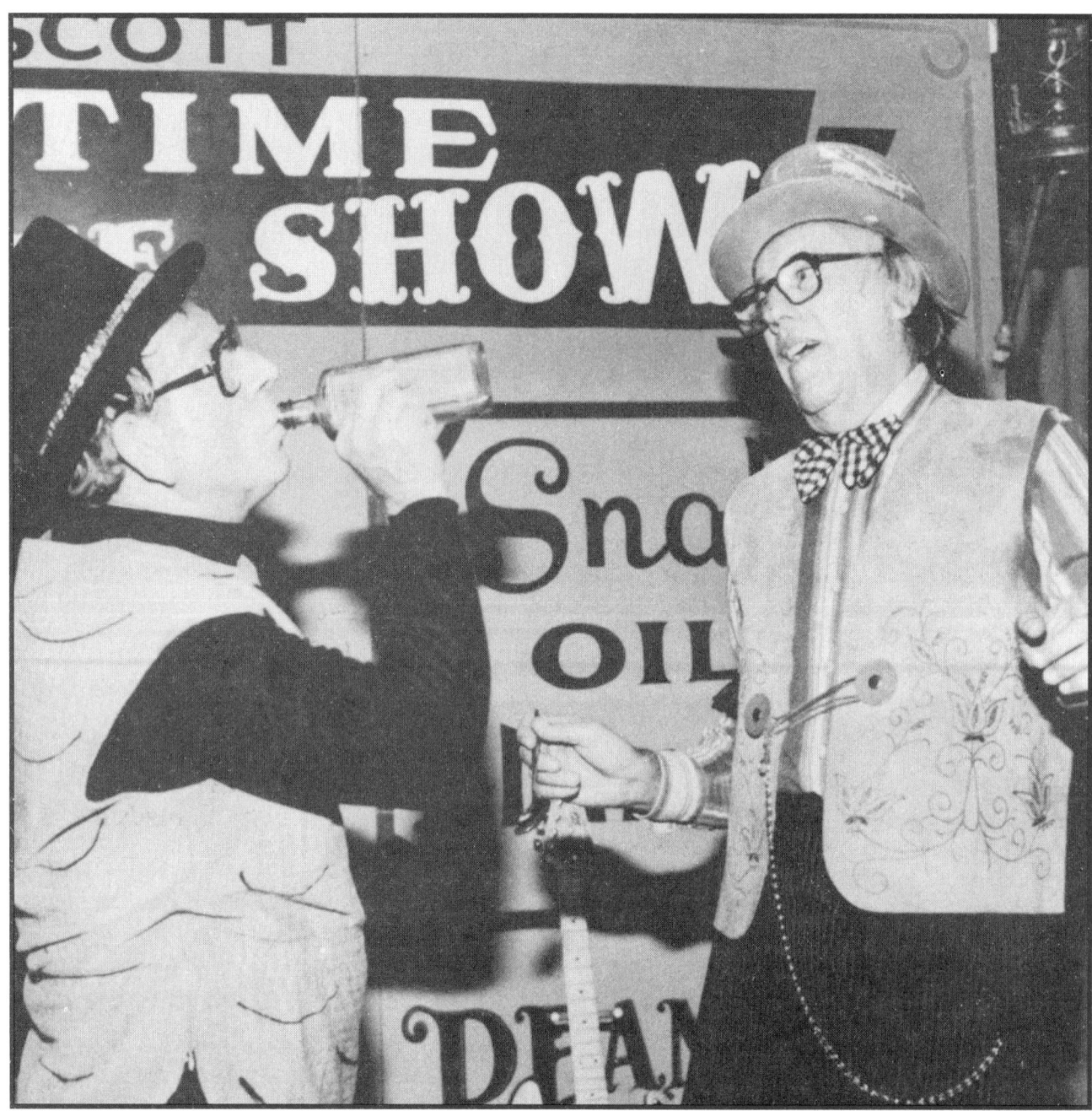

do—but he believed that his customers' faith in the product was half the cure. Still, he was a bit defensive about it. He spent years defending his business from the bad reputation it sometimes had because of unscrupulous shysters around the turn of the century who saw the medicine show as a way to make a quick buck.

In the old days, the medicine man mixed his own medicine in a porcelain tub in the back of the wagon and bottled it himself. The Pure Food and Drug Act of 1906 brought an end to that. There were still 200 medicine shows around the country at the time, but with the advent of stricter governmental regulation, the Depression, and the arrival of the greatest entertainer of all—television—they quickly fell by the wayside.

All, that is, except Doc Scott's show which became the second-longest-running traveling show, trailing only Ringling Brothers' Barnum & Bailey Circus.

Doc Scott's medicines came to be manufactured in a laboratory, though the ingredients hadn't changed. However, Doc Scott realized that he really sold two cures: a bottle of medicine, and an entertaining show where people could relax and have a good time.

The medicine show hadn't changed much since it began in 1890. Though performed in a school gym or community building instead of from the wagon or on an outdoor platform, the performers were much the same—jugglers, sharpshooters, unicyclists, ventriloquists, magicians and bluegrass musicians, including a musical saw act. Such shows provided the beginnings for country music, vaudeville, beauty contests and "amateur hour" productions.

At the radio station Tom was hired to add some of the picking and singing that was becoming so popular. Tom still sold his herbal medicine part time.

A few changes became necessary over the years. Admission was usually charged. Herb-O-Lac came in tablet form instead of liquid, and was not pushed as it once was. Snake Oil became the main product though its price increased from $1 to $5 a bottle.

Doc Scott appeared on *Entertainment Tonight, Nashville Now, The Today Show, Late Night with David Letterman, Late Night on NBC,* Walter Cronkite's *CBS News,* Charles Kuralt's *On the Road, CBS Sunday Morning,* a PBS special, on the BBC in London, Johnny Carson's *Tonight Show, The Oprah Winfrey Show* and many more.

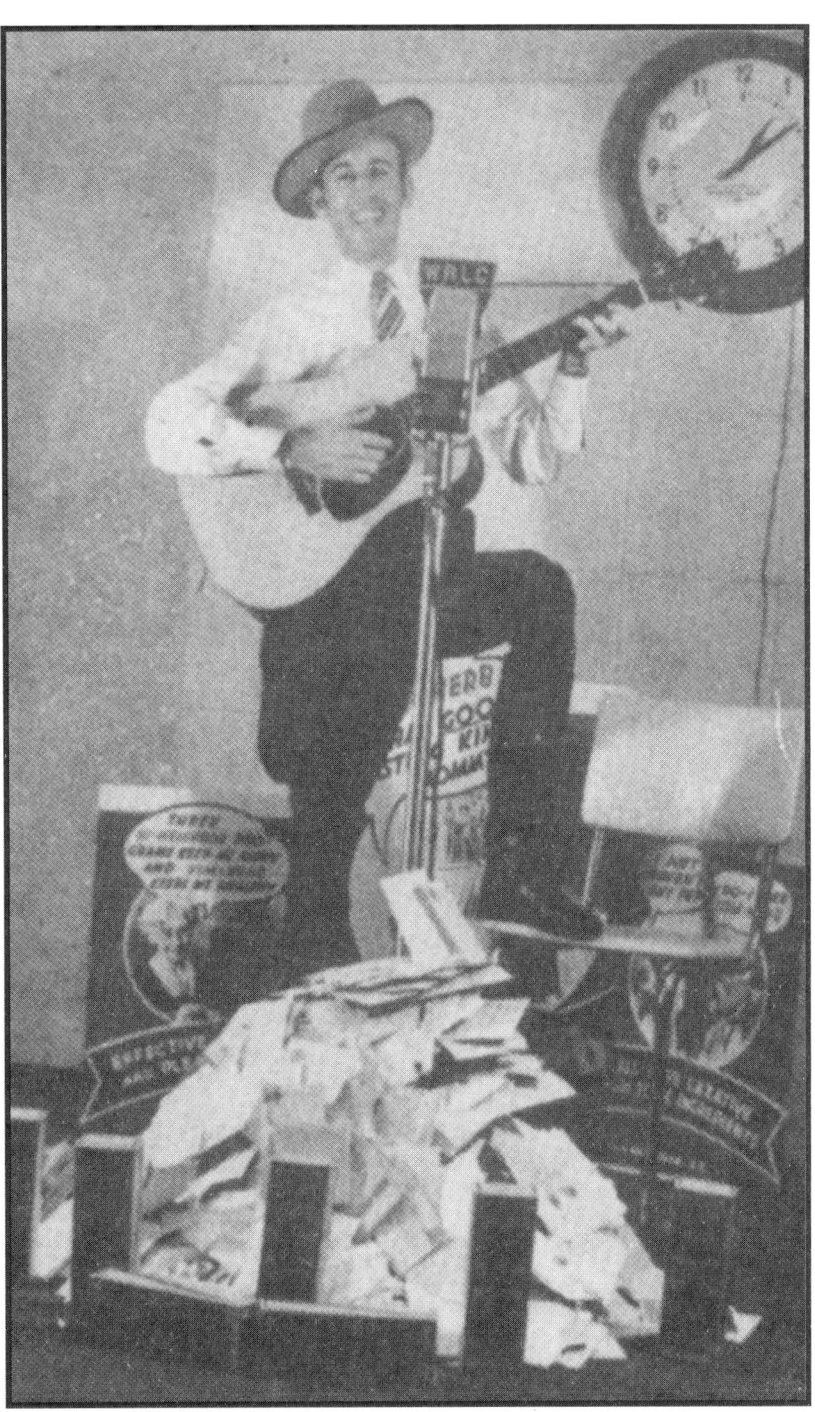

Tommy Scott during his first job after the Doc Chamberlain medicine show in 1936.

Looking at him, most people assumed him to be in his 50s. He was certainly a good advertisement for his products! He averaged a show a night, seven days a week, for 330 nights a year for over 50 years, playing mostly the small towns.

Doc Scott's was the last real old-time medicine show. ◆

Castor-Oil Days

By Marjorie H. Gardner

Mama was a worrier. Besides that, when she wanted something, she wanted it *now*. Her greatest worry and scantiest stock of patience concerned the matter of "regularity"—her own and that of my brother and me. "Have your bowels moved yet?" she would ask us each morning before our heads had barely left the pillow.

Our daily diet included Roman Meal mush, bran muffins, prunes and, since we lived in apple country, plenty of Delicious and Gravensteins. From this you know that we had the cleanest, emptiest insides of anyone in the state of California.

But if our answer to Mama's fateful question was "No" (we had been taught to always tell the truth), out came the big tablespoon and the bottle in which she currently rested her faith.

The first of these, Fletcher's Castoria, administered in our earliest childhood, was tolerable. Its slogan, "Children Cry For It" (or was it "Babies Cry For It"?), was exaggerated as far as we were concerned. At least we didn't cry *at* it, as at some later remedies.

Castoria was a gentle-acting brew, but Mama was looking for something more in the nature of TNT. Fletcher's, therefore, was soon discarded in favor of a concoction with a better track record.

Oh, lucky today's children who have never been forced to partake of the oil of the castor bean, *ricinus communis!* How our eyes bulged and crossed as the noxious, brimming spoon neared our tightly clenched lips. Rotten eggs, toadstools, *snakes* would have been more welcome! We were too young to know that anticipation merely prolongs the agony and, forgetting to keep our mouths closed, we screamed and hollered at our approaching doom.

As the noxious amber-green liquid trickled down our gagging throats, our whole being, our tonsils, our livers, cringed at the contact. Thick, viscous, it coated tongue, teeth and gullet with its unique flavor, leaving an aftertaste remembered to this day, some 60 years later.

When Mama heard about mixing the dose in orange juice, she tried to sell us on the tastiness of this beverage—unsuccessfully. A whole glass of the stuff, diluted though it was, meant that much more to get down.

When I suffered a long siege of mastoiditis in my ninth year and underwent the resulting mastoidectomy (unheard of in this day of wonder drugs), a sympathetic doctor introduced our mother to *cascara sagrada*. Compared to castor oil, this product was like chocolate milk. Papa had fond memories of cascara. It was made from buckthorn bark, and in his youth he had earned spending money by peeling back chittem (buckthorn) and selling it to the druggist in the city. Add to that the fact that Mama had so little trouble administering the stuff, and we were stuck with it for a while, although it always gave me stomach cramps. But life is no bowl of cherries, we were learning; it was a measure of one laxative or another.

When all else failed or when Mama was dissatisfied with the results, out came the contraption we dreaded even more than ricinus communis oil—the red rubber bag with the long, slender tubing and the black nozzle.

Then Mama discovered the ultimate remedy which shall remain nameless on these pages. Packaged in an ugly red-and-black can, it was the size of a horse pill. It was fast-acting, thorough and harsh enough to satisfy even her exacting standards.

In my 14th year I had the mumps—mumps and plenty of horse pills. One night after about my fifth rush to the bathroom, I blacked out and landed on the floor with a thud. I had been reading old-fashioned romances—*Graustark* and the like—in which the heroine often faints, much to the admiration of the hero, and me. To me, passing out was a thrilling event, one to be treasured and recorded in my diary: "April 9— First swoon." Mama failed to see it that way, and so ended the reign of the red-and-black can in our medicine chest.

That summer, when our city relatives came

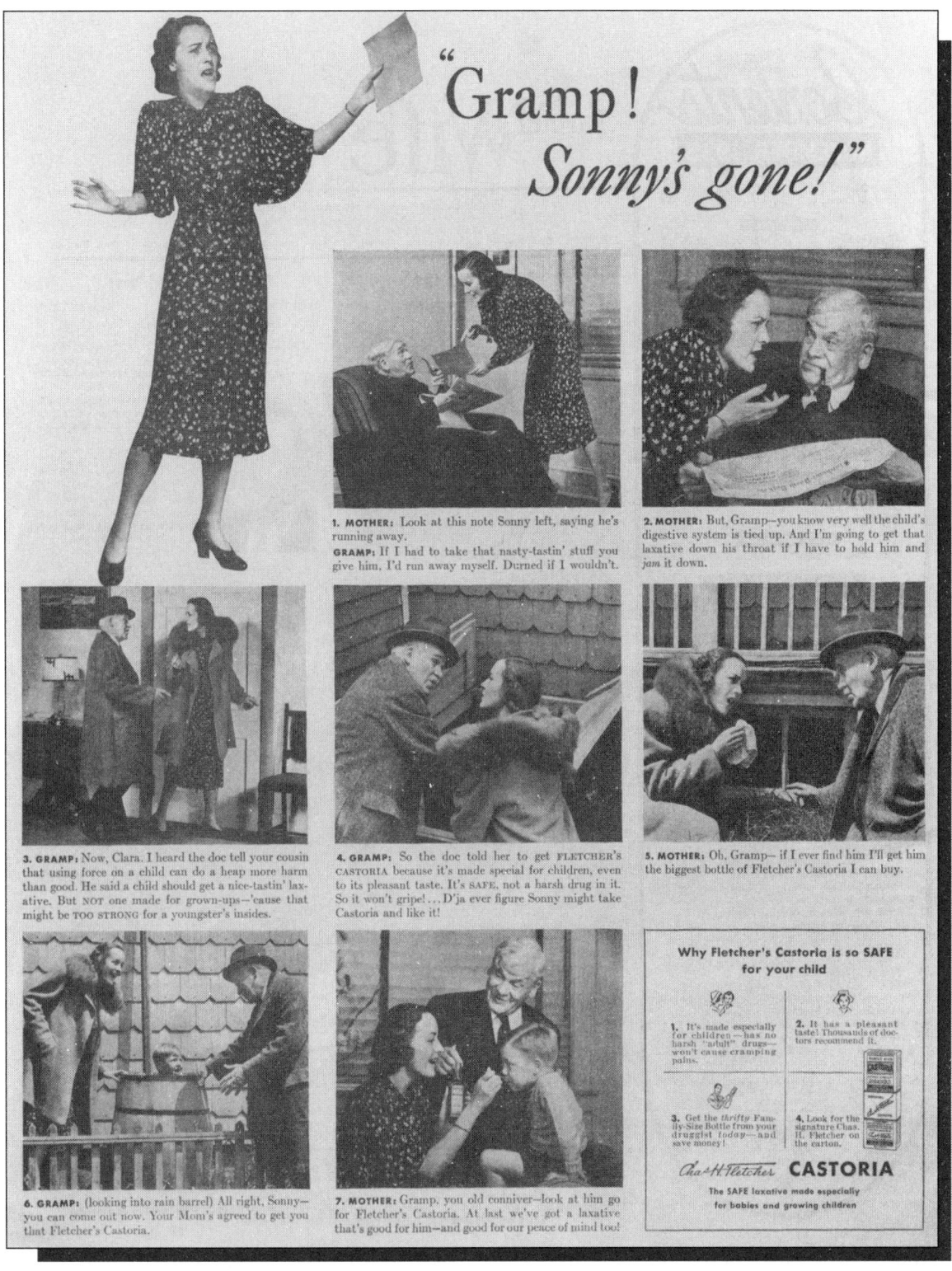

"Gramp! Sonny's gone!"

1. MOTHER: Look at this note Sonny left, saying he's running away.
GRAMP: If I had to take that nasty-tastin' stuff you give him, I'd run away myself. Durned if I wouldn't.

2. MOTHER: But, Gramp—you know very well the child's digestive system is tied up. And I'm going to get that laxative down his throat if I have to hold him and *jam* it down.

3. GRAMP: Now, Clara. I heard the doc tell your cousin that using force on a child can do a heap more harm than good. He said a child should get a nice-tastin' laxative. But NOT one made for grown-ups—'cause that might be TOO STRONG for a youngster's insides.

4. GRAMP: So the doc told her to get FLETCHER'S CASTORIA because it's made special for children, even to its pleasant taste. It's SAFE, not a harsh drug in it. So it won't gripe!...D'ja ever figure Sonny might take Castoria and like it!

5. MOTHER: Oh, Gramp— if I ever find him I'll get him the biggest bottle of Fletcher's Castoria I can buy.

6. GRAMP: (looking into rain barrel) All right, Sonny—you can come out now. Your Mom's agreed to get you that Fletcher's Castoria.

7. MOTHER: Gramp, you old conniver—look at him go for Fletcher's Castoria. At last we've got a laxative that's good for him—and good for our peace of mind too!

Why Fletcher's Castoria is so SAFE for your child

1. It's made especially for children—has no harsh "adult" drugs—won't cause cramping pains.

2. It has a pleasant taste! Thousands of doctors recommend it.

3. Get the *thrifty* Family-Size Bottle from your druggist *today*—and save money!

4. Look for the signature Chas. H. Fletcher on the carton.

Chas. H. Fletcher **CASTORIA**

The SAFE laxative made especially for babies and growing children

for their annual visit, their luggage contained a supply of Feen-A-Mint (they always learned about the latest developments before we did). However, Mama wouldn't let us use it—she took a dim view of gum chewing. "Makes you look like the old cow chewing her cud," she used to say.

So we finished our years at home with the old reliable—castor oil. I suspect now that the Roman Meal, the bran muffins and the rest of our country food was enough. Trouble was, Mama didn't know how much was enough—and she had to be sure! ◆

The Friday-Night Cure

By Joan Weston

My grandmother lived by this rule: A laxative once a week would cure almost anything. Every Friday at bedtime defenseless children were dosed with a tablespoon of castor oil. It did give us something to do on the weekend.

When I was 5 years old, my little brother and I had to stay with our grandparents while our father was in the hospital. I hadn't yet learned the names of the weekdays, but I soon learned to recognize Friday night.

On Friday night Grandma came into the bedroom with the castor oil, a spoon, and a couple of cookies. I cried, begged and gagged and only managed to swallow after she promised that the next time Grandpa went to town she would be sure to add Fletcher's Castoria to her shopping list. She said it was special for little kiddies, and that it didn't taste awful.

I forgot about it until Friday night came and Grandma came into the bedroom with a bottle of brown liquid and a spoon. I was apprehensive, but with a little coaxing I tasted the one drop she put on the spoon. It was good! The whole spoonful went down without so much as a tear.

A day or two later, my brother and I wandered into the pantry looking for cookies and we saw the new bottle of kiddie medicine on a shelf behind the door.

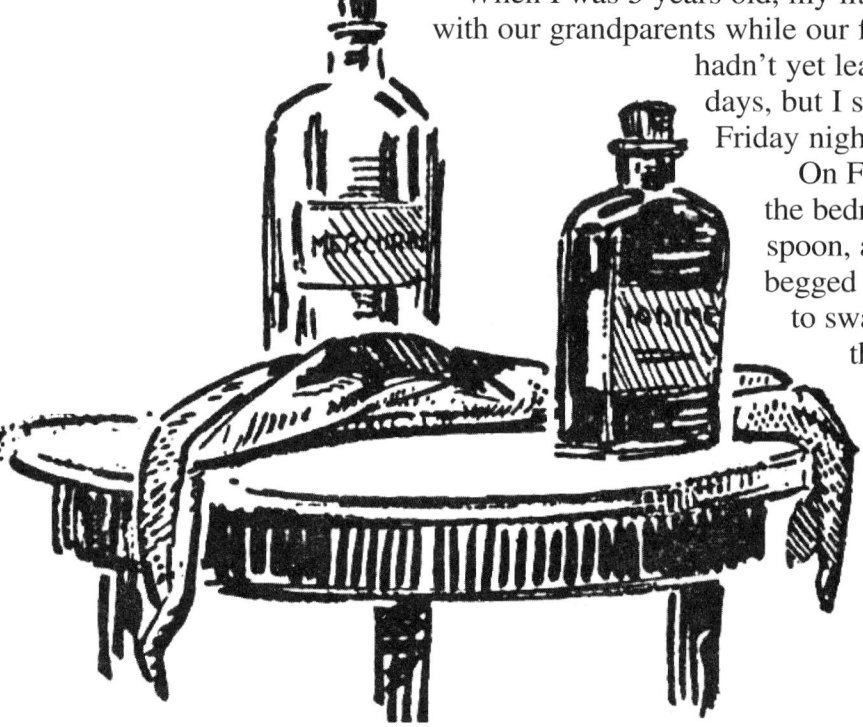

On Friday night Grandma came into the bedroom with the castor oil, a spoon, and a couple of cookies.

I had a taste and offered him one. He licked the top of the bottle and handed it back. I had another drink, and still another. The bottle was nearly empty when I put it back on the shelf and went to play.

Later that week I was playing by the chicken house when Grandpa drove the old car up to the back porch and got out, leaving the motor running. He ran behind the cellar and returned with the "company pot," put it between the seats, ran into the house, and returned with a roll of toilet tissue. (That was for company, too.)

I watched in awe. It was the only time I ever saw Grandpa touch a pot!

Grandpa ran toward the barn for a last-minute check on the stock, and I went into the house to see what was happening. Grandma was standing in front of the dresser, pinning on her hat. She was wearing her good navy blue dress.

"Are we going to town?" I asked excitedly.

"Yes," she answered, her voice trembling. "We have to take you to the doctor."

"Me? To the doctor? Why? I'm not sick," I protested.

"You may not be sick now, but I'm afraid you're going to be soon. That Castoria bottle is nearly empty."

"I didn't mean to drink that much, but it was good," I told her.

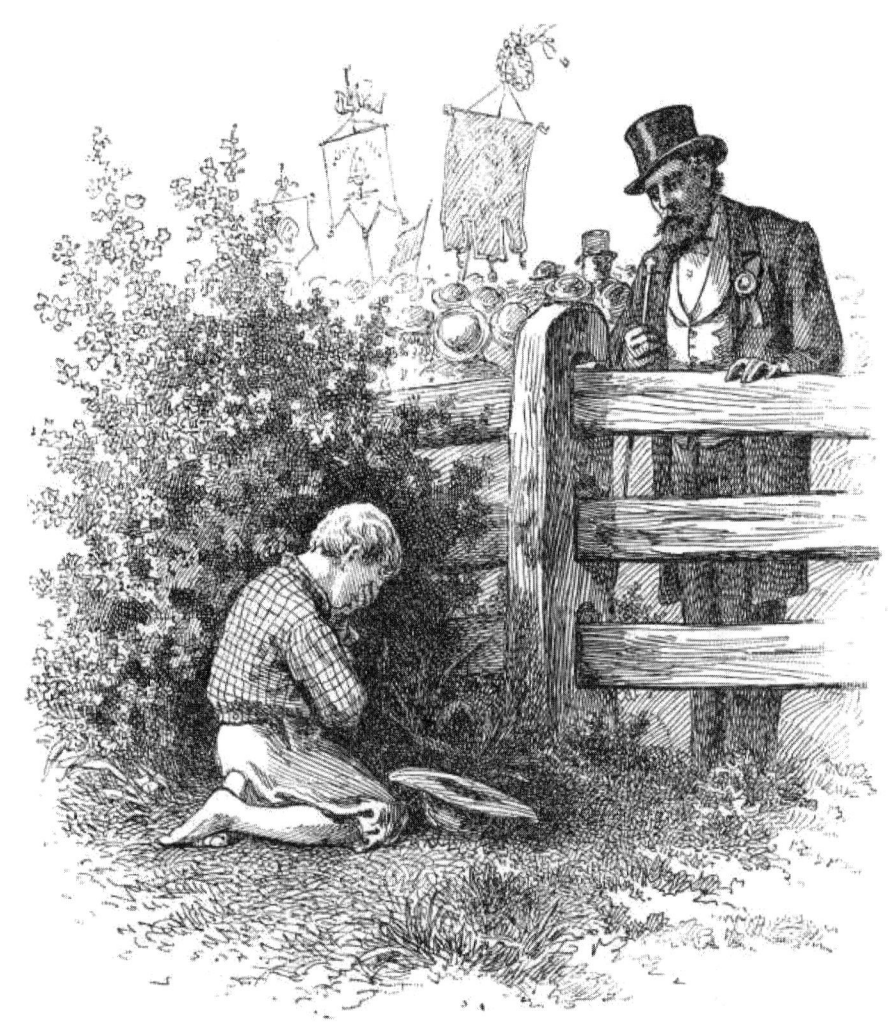

"We have to take you to the doctor," she answered, her voice trembling. "You may not be sick now, but I'm afraid you're going to be soon. That Castoria bottle is nearly empty."

"Where was I when you drank it?" she asked.

"I don't know; it was so long ago, I forgot," I said.

"You mean you didn't drink it today? When did you drink it? Do you remember?"

"Several days ago," I replied.

"Didn't you have a problem or a sore tail?"

"No, I just felt like me," I said.

Grandma took her hat off. Grandpa moved the car, and I never got another Friday-night laxative again. ◆

Grandma Was Another Lydia Pinkham?

By Julie Marshall

Over 20 years ago, an article in the newspaper reported that after 87 years, the Lydia Pinkham Medicine Co. had been sold. This great old lady reminded me of another great old lady, my grandmother.

Like my grandmother, Lydia Pinkham was a Quaker. And like my grandmother, she practiced medicine without a license. By "practiced medicine" I mean that Grandma concocted home remedies to cure specific ills. But here the similarities cease. Mrs. Pinkham's remedy was for certain female complaints, whereas my grandmother's cures took care of the entire family, male and female. She never tried to sell them, nor did any contain alcohol. When my brother, Paul, and I were growing up, our family never had a doctor. We had Grandma.

Like my grandmother, Lydia Pinkham was a Quaker. And like my grandmother, she practiced medicine without a license.

The most commonly employed remedy was for a cold. This particular cure did not originate with Grandma, but she certainly took advantage of it. If the cold was in my chest, she swabbed me with lard and wrapped my neck in a flannel rag and secured it with a large safety pin. (Mother used to insist that it should be red flannel, but Grandma said, "Pshaw, Lizzie, that's superstitious nonsense," and went on with her doctoring.) If coughing ensued, she mixed a little butter and sugar to soothe the throat. Bed rest accompanied this "medication." The whole treatment was probably as effective as anything science has discovered to date.

Lard was an ingredient in another of Grandma's home remedies. She mixed it with sulfur and spread it between our fingers when we came home with "the itch." Whether it cured it or not is questionable, but it certainly eased the itching. It is significant that many of today's preparations for pruritis still contain sulfur.

In the summer, happiness was going barefoot. This, however, was not without hazards. Once I stepped on a rusty nail, receiving a horrible puncture wound in my foot. Today a child would be sped to the family doctor for a booster shot of anti-tetanus serum. But in those days, my grandmother calmly went about her business mixing a bread-and-milk poultice. She soaked bread in warm milk until it was of proper consistency and applied it to the foot which was then swathed in clean cloths. The idea was to draw out the poison. It must have worked—either that, or there were no tetanus germs lurking to pounce on my wound, for in any case, lockjaw never developed.

Children's pleasures were simple then and most were homemade. We made stilts, tin can horseshoes, slingshots and bows and arrows. We whittled our arrows out of old shingles using a butcher knife. I was 6 years old and busily notching the end of a completed arrow when the blade slipped, cutting my left index finger to the bone.

Was I rushed to the plastic surgeon to repair the laceration with the obviously necessary half-dozen (or more) sutures? You bet your bottle of Bromo-Seltzer I wasn't. Grandmother bound the wound tightly with a clean rag to hold the severed edges together. Then she had me lie down and covered me with a blanket to keep me warm and quiet,

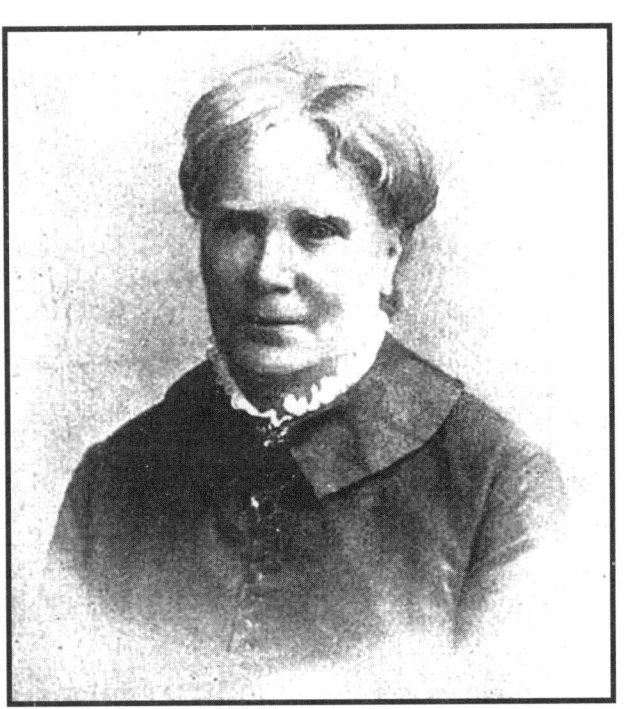

seeming to know instinctively about shock. My finger healed with minimal scarring and no sequelae—except for the spanking Grandma administered for using the forbidden butcher knife.

One day Paul discovered a bottle of castor oil on the top shelf in the kitchen. We dared each other to try it. Paul went first. When he tried it, the smell sickened me to the extent that I couldn't keep my end of the bargain. Fortunately, we never had to take it. I think it must have been used to oil the sewing machine. Grandma had a much better remedy than castor oil.

Every now and then she took out her wooden bowl and her rocker-type chopper and chopped up a batch of walnuts, dates and raisins. She formed the mixture into balls a little larger than a marble, rolled them in powdered sugar and stored them away to mellow and be ready for one purpose only.

However, my brother and I discovered that they were quite tasty. We ignored their designated purpose and helped ourselves whenever we craved a little taste treat. This had no adverse effect on our elimination. Perhaps Grandma was only kidding herself with this remedy.

We were inclined to try to kid Grandma, too, if we couldn't get the goodies any other way. We would double over and groan, holding our stomachs. If Grandmother suspected us of malingering, she threatened dire consequences with a horrible contraption of tubes and a rubber bag. Her threat induced an instant and miraculous cure. Grandmother was blind, but it was nearly impossible to fool her, as she had all her other senses working double for her.

She, along with Mrs. Pinkham, has gone to that big pharmacy in the sky, where no doubt she is stirring up the Lord knows what heavenly brew for ailing angels. Those of us left below must now be satisfied with the corner drugstore. With all deference to Grandma, the corner pharmacy is much preferred over home remedies. We were probably lucky that we were never seriously ill.

Grandma's remedies are never used anymore, but Lydia's magic potion, somewhat modified as to contents, can still be found on the apothecary's shelf, and it still claims to bring relief to women from certain discomforts peculiar to their gender.

As one druggist remarked, "There is a small percentage of alcohol in it, so it at least makes you feel better while you have it." ◆

First Hospital in a Cow Town

By Jack Jennings

O ur town's emergency treatment was rendered in the offices of Drs. Rivers, Brinson and Gieger. Critical cases were then taken to the Orange General Hospital in Orlando, Fla. Other illnesses were treated during office calls or when the doctor visited the patient's home. That was the way it had been for years. Folks paid with eggs, chicken, produce, fresh meat, cash or nothing at all. The doctors rendered assistance at any hour, night or day, and were highly respected citizens of the county.

When these doctors retired in the late '20s, a new doctor converted the large, two-story Penton residence into Kissimmee Hospital. In a few months, his practice had grown and he was joined by another doctor from a large northern city who was immediately impressed by the rural cow country.

This Dr. Jewel was a small young man, slight of build and with a pale complexion, in considerable contrast to most of the large, raw-boned, swarthy cowmen and commercial fisherman of the area—especially Uncle Walt Bronson. The rancher stood about 6 feet 3 inches in his stocking feet and wore the old knee-length laced leather boots and a black 10-gallon Stetson.

One cold November day Uncle Walt rode out to check some of his cattle and forgot to tie his wagon slicker behind his saddle. It rained hard and when he returned that evening he was soaked to the skin. The next morning he was "under the weather" with chills and fever. Aunt Sue sent him to bed and administered doses of a cure-all remedy concocted from hot honey, lemonade, baking soda and 'shine whiskey.

In a few days Walt was up and around and feeling well enough to go into town for supplies. Aunt Sue told him to stop by the doctor's office at the hospital and get a prescription if further medication was needed. Uncle Walt had not been in the new hospital or met the new Dr. Jewel, so he decided to follow Aunt Sue's

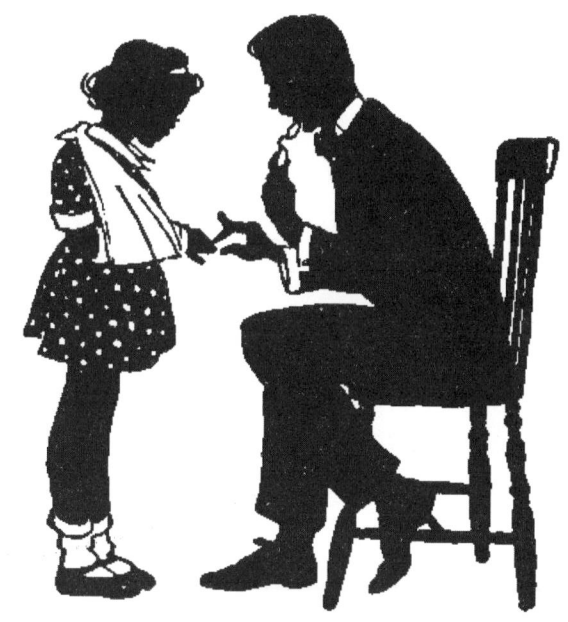

instructions (which was always the path of least resistance).

Uncle Walt walked into the waiting room of the Kissimmee Hospital and took a seat to wait his turn. The nurse came in shortly with Dr. Jewel and said, "Next patient!" Uncle Walt stood up, placed his *Kissimmee Valley Gazette* on the table and started into the doctor's office. Dr. Jewel was standing in the doorway, all decked out in high-heeled cowboy boots, new Levi pants and a hand-tooled leather belt with a big silver buckle.

Uncle Walt took note of this stranger with a quick glance and sat back down. "Pardon me, son," he drawled, "you go right on in first to see the doctor. You look like you need him a darn sight worse than I do!"

Aunt Sue's Flu Remedy

1 teaspoon baking soda
1 tablespoon honey
Juice of 1 lemon
⅓ cup 'shine whiskey

Mix all ingredients in a pint fruit jar filled with boiling-hot water. Drink while hot and stay in bed. ◆

Homemade Salve

By Norma Ulmer

The recipe for homemade salve has come down through many generations. When the supply was getting low, someone usually announced that she would make a new cooking.

It began with a trip to the fields for a handful of stalks from the elderberry bush. The outer layer of the stalk was scraped away. Then, with a piece of broken pottery, the next layer was shredded until the correct amount was obtained. Next was a trip to the drugstore. Here equal amounts of alum, resin, beeswax and saffron blossoms were obtained. Now came a stop at the butcher shop for several pounds of mutton tallow and pure lard.

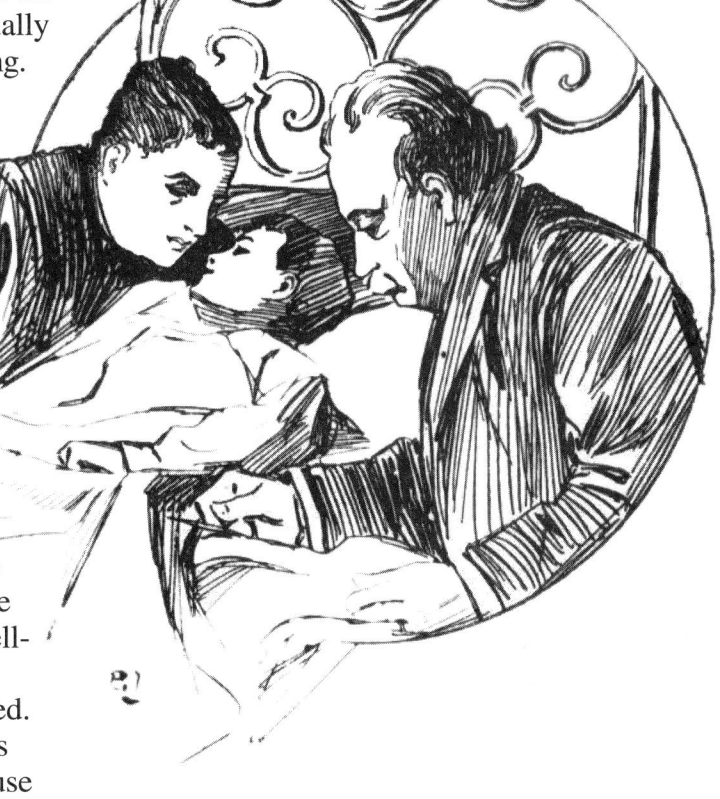

All of the ingredients were put in a large skillet and placed on the wood-burning stove to simmer. It was mixed and stirred until well-blended, then strained through a piece of cheesecloth, poured into small jars and sealed.

Each household in the neighborhood was given a jar. One jar was kept in the barn to use on the horses' aching shoulders and on the teats of the cows when they became sore from wading through mud or being scratched by briars or barbed wire.

In the house it was used on any open sore. If a child stepped on a rusty nail or got a thorn in the foot, Mother put a lump of salve on the wound and bandaged it tightly. It drew out all impurities, even foreign objects like thorns and bits of glass. It healed from the inside out.

One time I fell on the schoolhouse porch and ran a nail head in my knee. Mother applied a bandage of homemade salve and it quickly healed. I still have the scar.

My grandson and his wife have a new baby who developed diaper rash. When it did not heal from the doctor's prescription, Jim said, "Try some of Grandma's salve." It healed nicely.

Now Jim is a "convert" and says he will make the next cooking!

Homemade Salve

In late summer, get several stems of an elderberry bush. Remove the outer layer. With a dull knife, scrape the second layer until you have the desired amount. Then, in a large, heavy skillet mix:

    ½ cup shaved elder
    ½ cup beeswax
    ½ cup rosin
    ½ cup mutton tallow
    ½ cup saffron blossoms
    ½ cup alum
    6 cups unsalted lard

Mix and stir until thoroughly cooked. Strain and put into jars. ◆

Spring Tonic

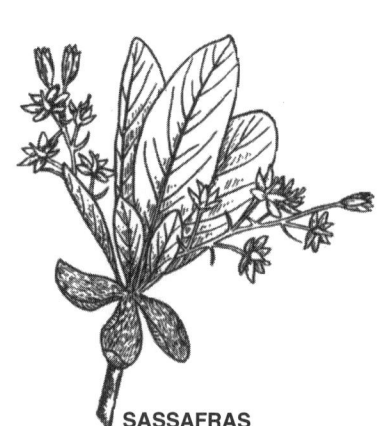

SASSAFRAS

By Francis Sculley

In my childhood, one of the sure signs of spring was the appearance of the Seneca lady with her immense basket loaded with strips of sassafras tied in bundles so uniform, one would swear they had been machined. She took her place in front of the Commercial National Bank as busy townspeople passed in and out through the swinging doors.

Sassafras is now sold in supermarkets, packaged in cellophane bags and drier than a Kansas dust storm. But thousands of Americans still look forward to their annual spring tonic—sassafras tea, one of the hundreds of contributions made by the first Americans.

While known as a shrub in northern parts, the cousin of the mountain laurel occasionally soars to 40 feet in southern states. The twigs and buds of *Sassafras albidium* provide the basic ingredient for the Creole delicacy known as gumbo.

Thousands of Americans still look forward to their annual spring tonic—sassafras tea, one of the hundreds of contributions made by the first Americans.

In Pennsylvania's northern tier of counties, the leaf-shedding shrub rarely attains a height over 8 feet—usually closer to 4 feet—as it grows in borders of woods, old fields which were once pastureland, and along the fencerows.

Branches of sassafras are yellowish green to red, smooth, or downy like sumac. The leaves are alternate, oval or elliptic, and often with multiple lobes. Buds and twigs are spicy and aromatic when crushed, and the greenish yellow flowers, which appear in clusters, bloom from March to May depending on the locale. The oval, dark blue fruit bears a single seed and is borne on red, club-shaped stalks. A cousin to the blueberry, it bears its fruit from June to October but is usually considered a fall berry in northern climes.

The roots of the fragrant shrub are uncovered, and strips 6 to 8 inches in length are cut from the tough wood. After a thorough washing, it is easy to see the pink and white inner bark, as spongy as rubber, from which a fiery oil is made to flavor candies and medicine.

Pioneer families in Vermont and New Hampshire produced aromatic soaps from hog fat and lye, and scented with sassafras oil.

But it was the tea made from the dried bark that made the plant popular. The Baroness Reidesel, whose husband was an officer in Burgoyne's ill-fated 1777 invasion of New York, makes mention of sassafras tea, and it is believed that Lord Balcarres and General Fraser learned to like the hot, spicy drink which was introduced to them by the Tory irregulars who accompanied the redcoat army.

The shrub, as American as succotash, is found from southwestern Maine westward to Michigan and south to Florida and Texas, being particularly abundant in the Allegheny Mountain range of Pennsylvania and New York.

Its fruits are eaten by wild birds, including grouse and wild turkey, and in the grasslands of southern Pennsylvania and Ohio, bobwhite quail thrive on them. The twigs are eaten by deer, rabbits and that most voracious of all rodents, the porcupine.

Although the plentiful shrub is unknown by most younger Americans today, earlier generations still fondly remember gathering this aromatic root from the hills. ◆

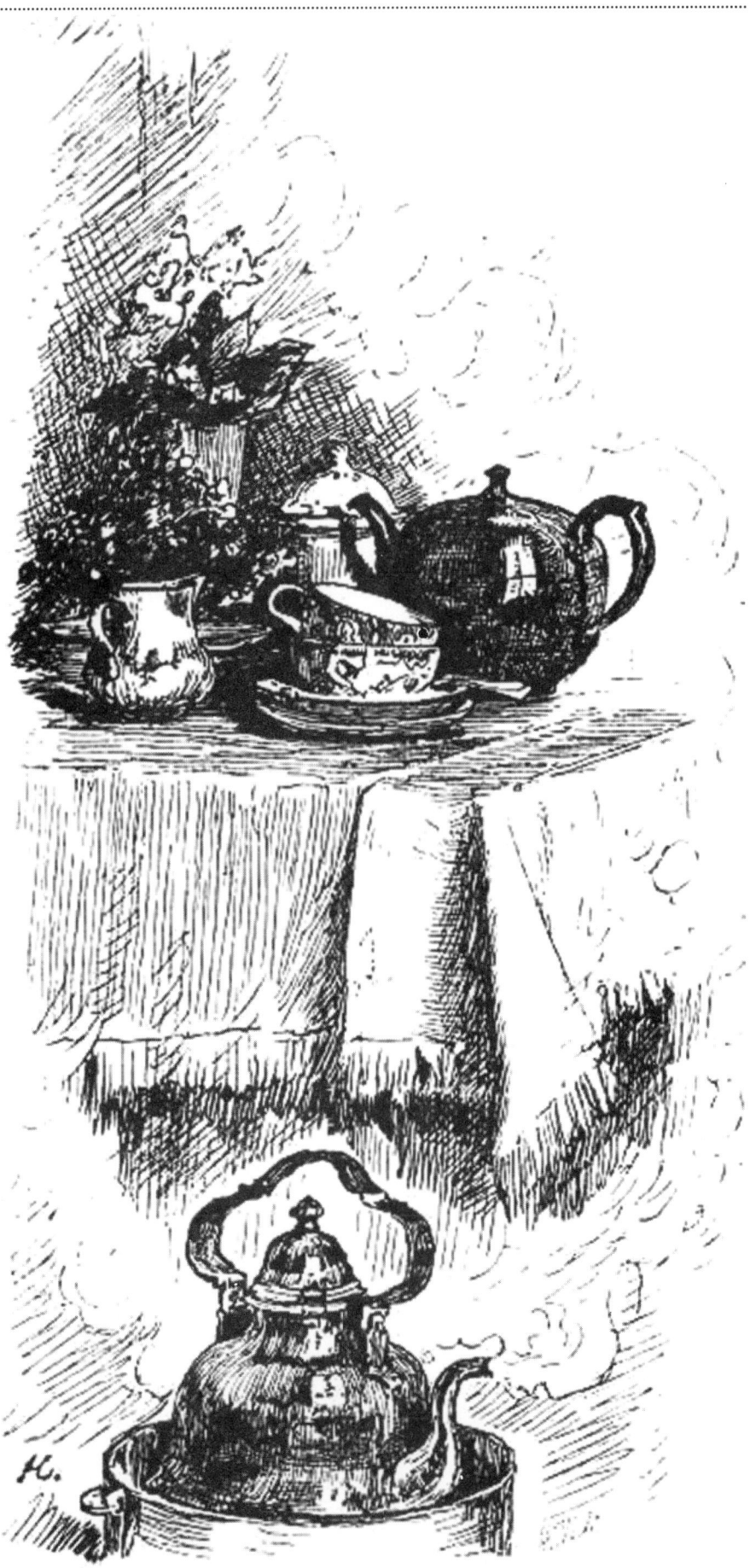

Home Remedies

Ground Itch

When my 3-year old brother, Roger, had ground itch, I was elected to scratch his toes. Ground itch is like ringworm and usually comes from wading in mud puddles. Mama put turpentine on them to stop the itching. I got the bottle and put some more on his toes, then got the box of matches so I could warm the turpentine to make his feet stop itching faster. Roger's foot caught fire and became a blaze. I grabbed a towel and put the fire out. It didn't blister the foot, but it sure cured the ground itch. I didn't have to scratch any more toes—but I surely didn't try that remedy again.

Jessie Hightower

Ringworm

Mix axle grease with a good amount of tobacco juice. Spread on a piece of cloth and tape in place over the ringworm. This is an old and dependable remedy.

Alma Holten

For Cold On the Lungs

½ cup lard
5 cents' worth of gum camphor
1 tablespoon turpentine
1 tablespoon coal oil
5 cents' worth of laudanum

Fry lard with gum camphor until dissolved; place in a can which has a tight cover. When the mixture is in the can and while it is still warm, add the turpentine, coal oil and laudanum.

To use, spread the mixture on flannel and put on chest.

Ruth Cox Anderson

Cough Syrup

When I was a child, I remember my mother making a cough syrup for us using:

    ½ cup honey
    ¼ cup brandy

Juice of 1 lemon

Bring it to a boil and boil for just a short while. Let cool and store in a covered jar. Take 1–2 teaspoons as needed for a bad cough.

I used this on my own children as they were growing up and usually have some made and on hand yet, especially during the winter.

M.B. Lewiston

Old-time remedy recipes for ground itch, ringworm, a cold on the lungs and cough syrup.

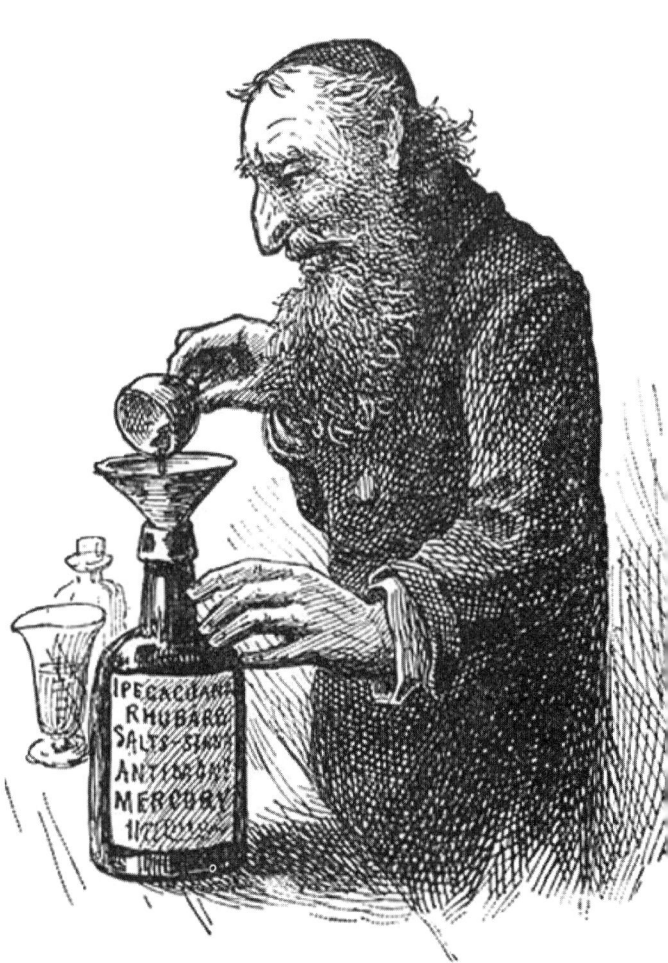

Old Remedies

By Marie Lundgren

I smile to think of what they used
To help us kids survive,
But I am going on 69
And very much alive.
My sorest throats were eased, and I
Still hold no bit of rancor
To think of sucking sugar lumps
With a drop or two of camphor.

And camphor mixed with goose grease for
A winter chest congestion;
Baking soda cleaned my teeth
And helped my indigestion.

Because of Mother's tender heart
I hereby sing a "Gloria!"
She never gave me castor oil,
Just syrupy Castoria.

Salt for all mosquito bites,
Cobwebs on the scratches,
The sickroom fumigated with
Our sulphur kitchen matches.
Somehow there's quite a bunch of us
That never had a shot,
But here we are, still kicking and
Enjoying it a lot.

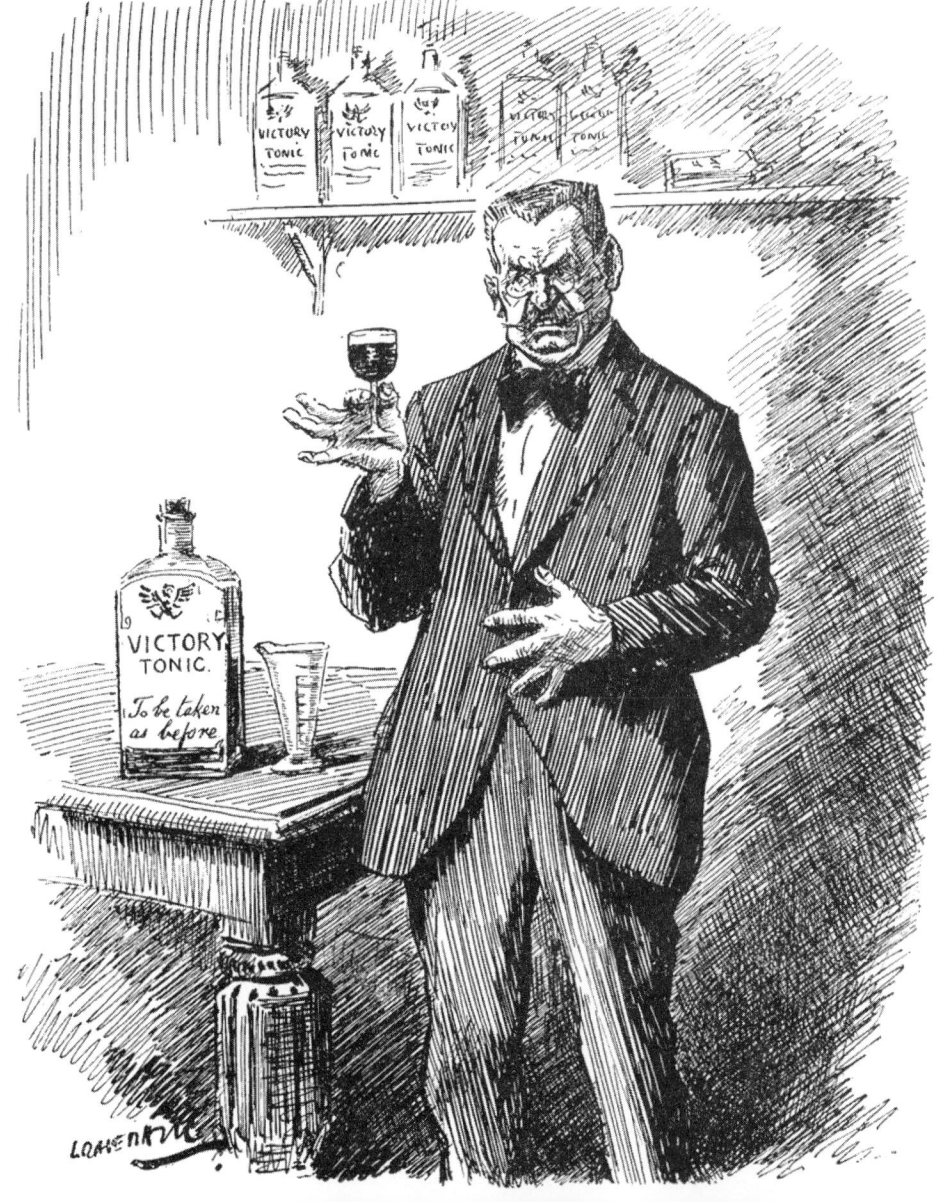

Mother's Guru Remedy—Vaseline

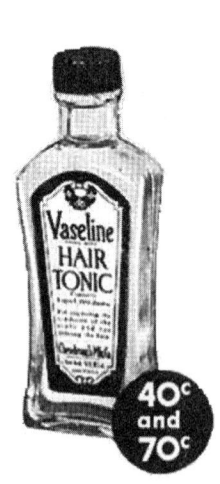

By Florine Cherwin

Lydia E. Pinkham was my mother's cure-all for women's discomforts, and some green drops took the place of today's antacids. Molasses-like cough syrup was "good for you" because it took the hack out, and mustard plaster soothed an aching back and rejuvenated sore muscles. But the big genie of them all was Vaseline. Mother called it "Old Faithful."

With it she removed burrs from the cat's hair, which also gave him a licking good time and rid him of hairballs. Applied to small cuts before bandaging, Vaseline "held the cut together." It polished my patent-leather shoes, softened callouses, got the red out of chapped hands and offered instant therapy to bumps and bruises. Mother even used it on creaky or stubborn door hinges, including the oven door on our long-legged gas stove.

When lice got into my hair after a visit to Grandfather's pigeon coop, my frantic mother immediately shampooed my hair with Fels-Naphtha soap and then rubbed Vaseline all over my head to "take out the soap smell and bring back the natural oils." An Ivory Soap shampoo followed. No louse could survive that decontamination.

At an age when movie stars were goddesses to be emulated, I tried to copy the slick hairstyles of Norma Shearer, Pola Negri and Clara Bow. Since the stars I admired were brunettes and I was blond, I spread Vaseline over my hair to darken and smooth it back, and then brought forth spit curls over my forehead and cheeks. I felt sophisticated and proud as I sneaked out of the house to meet my friend who had used soap and water to form her spit curls. We looked gorgeous, but not for long. Sister Reihnfreda sent us home. My astounded but not intimidated mother took over from there, but before she grounded me, she said, "… And don't blame it on Old Faithful."

Having grown up with this mind-set, my own medicine cabinet, while reflecting modern, more sophisticated remedies, still contains a jar of Vaseline. My children grew up with the same respect for their grandmother's cure-all. They felt very comfortable with its remedial qualities and we too called it Old Faithful.

My 6-year-old son was playing with a spring-operated toy when it suddenly let loose and pulled the skin from his palm. My panic subsided

> *The big genie of all the home cures was Vaseline. Mother called it "Old Faithful."*

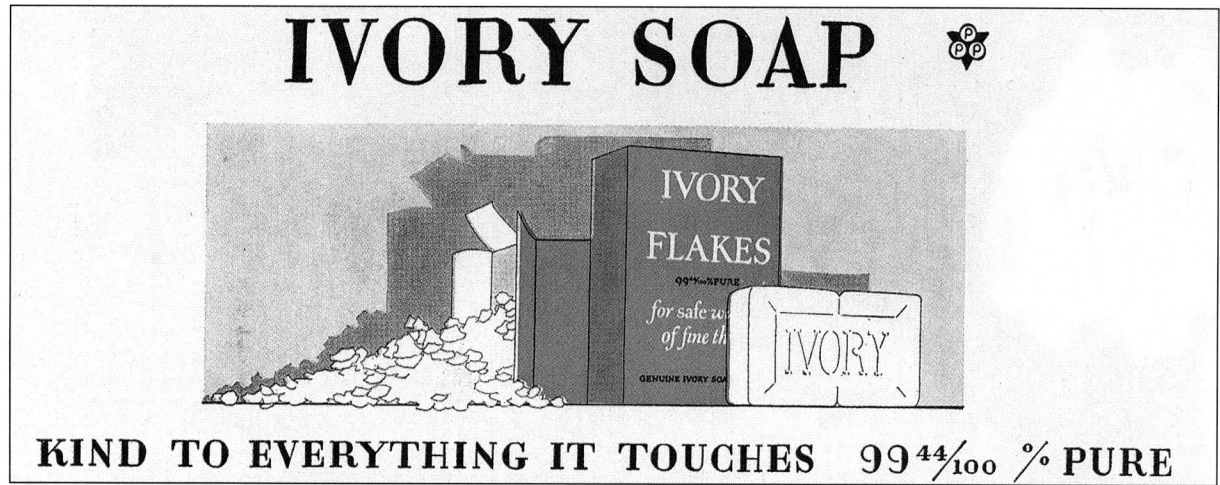
when I thought of Old Faithful. I cleansed the wound and put Vaseline on the bandage before wrapping it around his hand. When we got to the doctor for a tetanus shot, he approved my first-aid. I think that even if my mother had known about tetanus shots, she would have relied on Vaseline.

Petroleum jelly removes everything: mascara, scuff marks on the floor, and adhesive residue from labels on plastic and glass bottles. When complimented on my complexion, I give credit to the Vaseline I slathered on my face every night. It was also my mother's beauty treatment and she, too, had lovely skin.

I once saw her stem a kitchen ant invasion by covering their entrance and exit areas with Vaseline and then wiping off the excess. Now I do the same. I prefer not to use chemically treated products because of my visiting grandchildren, so I use a toothpick to force Vaseline into the openings the ants find so appealing. There is hardly any mess.

My most rewarding experience with Vaseline occurred when my youngest son received a chameleon as a gift from his aunt. The 7-year-old was ecstatic. I didn't share his enthusiasm, but he promised to feed it and tend to its needs. So Cammy, as he named him, became part of the household. I even let the creature lie on my arm to show my son I wasn't chicken. Cammy sunned himself (we assumed it was a he) on my rubber plant, changed colors and hopped about on my curtains.

All went well until the day Cammy was nowhere to be found. We searched the kitchen without results. Then I opened the door to the basement—and felt a crunch. I gently removed the tiny, limp body.

"Is he dead?" my son asked. There was a hole where Cammy's left eye had been and a trickle of blood. His skin was gray and his body lifeless. "Let's take him to the doctor for some penicillin," pleaded my son.

Knowing Cammy had joined his ancestors, I soothed my son. "Let's try first aid. Get Old Faithful."

I applied a blob over the hole in Cammy's head and gently laid him at the base of my rubber plant, explaining that an injury causes shock, and that's why Cammy was so still. I couldn't admit that it was all over for his pet.

After about three days I figured it was about time to flush Cammy or bury him in the back yard and lovingly tell my son that his pet's injury had been too great. But before I could prime myself to break the news, my son burst in. "Mom, Cammy moved," he reported. "He's feeling better. Come and see!"

And there was our injured chameleon playing hide-and-go-seek over the curtains. His skin was emerald, and though the hole in his head remained, there was still the glint of a hidden eye, giving him a clownish, rakish look that made us laugh. My son invited his friends to view his comical chameleon and I became known as the mother who revived reptiles—the James Herriott of the neighborhood.

I like to think that Old Faithful played a role in Cammy's survival. My mother, however, would not have had a single doubt. ◆

A Lovely Kettle of Tea

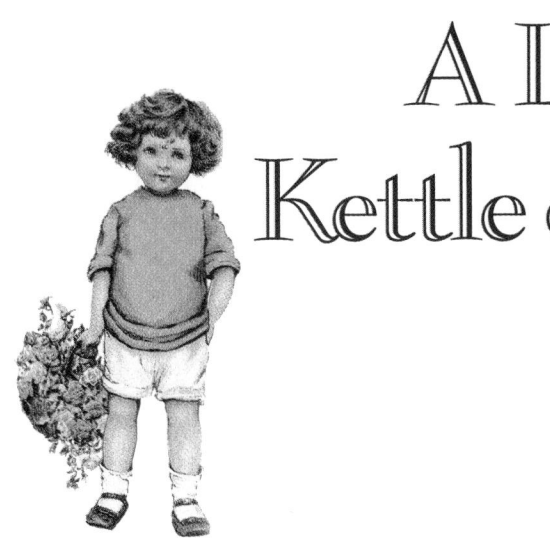

By Lucy Tharp

I recently read about the ancient Babylonian custom of placing a sick person in the marketplace in a position where everyone passing could see him. Passersby were obliged to ask the sick person how he felt and what he had done to improve his condition. Then they would offer suggestions to aid in the person's recovery.

When someone recommended a cure that had been successful before, the ill person was immediately taken home and treated with this remedy. The knowledge of the herbal remedies spread and, thus, the art of folk medicine was born.

As a young girl growing up in a mountainous section of Tennessee, I had the pleasure of being associated with two people who practiced the art of folk healing extensively.

Adam and Zora Duncan lived in a log house on a rundown hill farm. They were not much for socializing; indeed, they were regarded by their neighbors as being "quire" ("queer"). In the vernacular of the mountains, this term was ascribed to those whose customs deviated from what was considered to be the norm. People did pay frequent visits to the Duncan house, but not for social calls. Zora Duncan was highly regarded for the herb teas she prepared in her home.

My first encounter with the Duncans was accidental. I was picking blackberries along the fencerows of the Duncan place one day when, quite unexpectedly, I looked up to see Adam and Zora standing over me.

I expected to be sent packing. I had heard that the Duncans looked with a jaundiced eye upon intruders. Surprisingly, however, they put me at ease by showing me where the best berries grew.

Then they explained that they were gathering mullion leaves for tonic. I was literally dumbfounded when Zora asked me if I would like to accompany her on one of her herb-gathering expeditions. I replied that I would ask Mother, although I didn't have much hope of receiving her permission.

Several times during the next few days I tried to broach the subject tentatively with Mother by asking her about the Duncans. Each time she cut the conversation short by explaining that Adam and Zora Duncan were "quire" people and didn't like being bothered by company.

I wanted very much to learn about herbs and remedies, but I knew better than to argue with my parents.

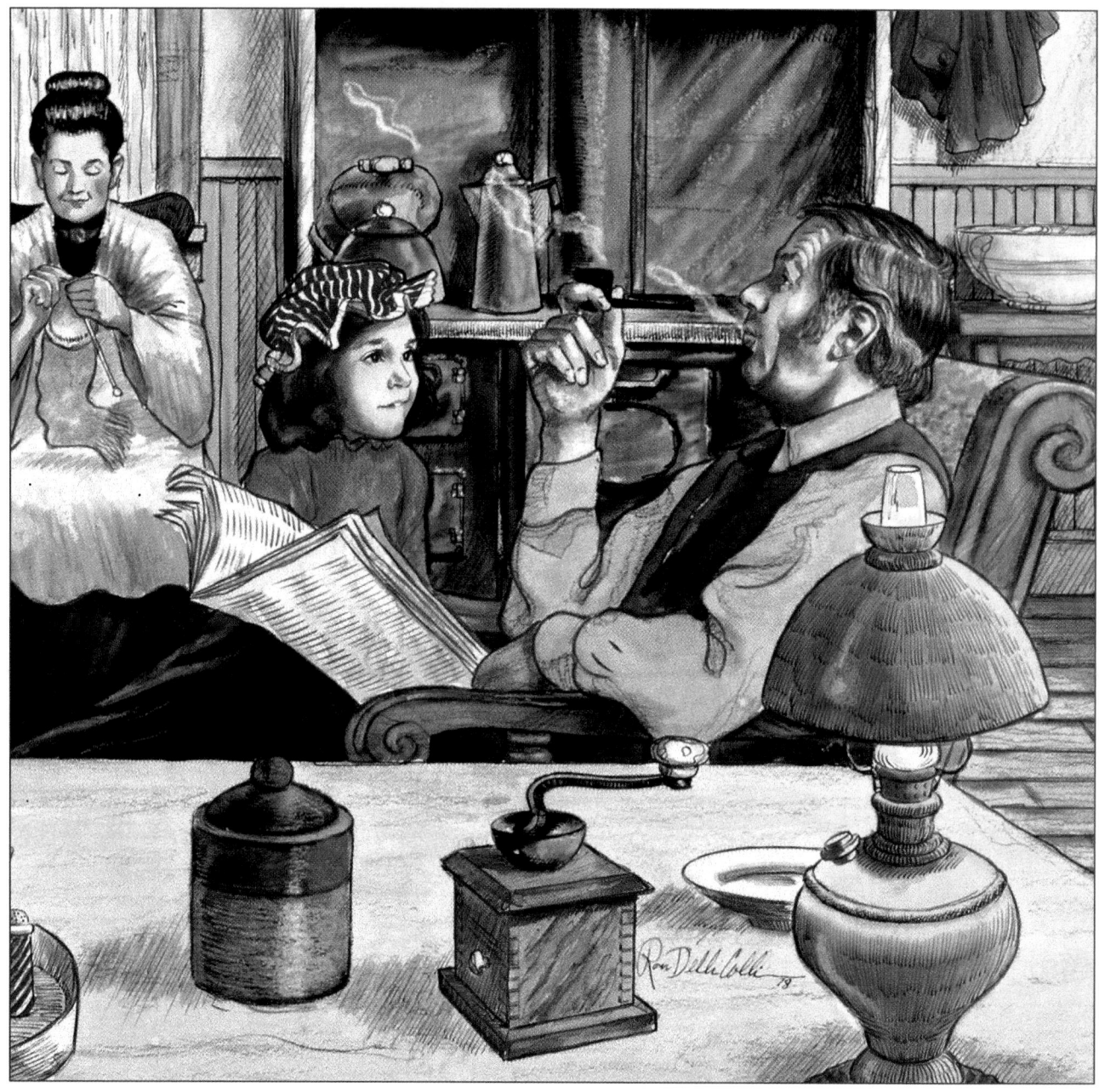

I wanted very much to learn about herbs and remedies, but I knew better than to argue with my parents. I had just about abandoned hope when, oddly enough, I received help from an unexpected source. One morning as we were clearing the breakfast table, there was a knock at our front door. Our early morning visitor proved to be Adam Duncan.

The Duncans raised very little in the way of food. They depended primarily on their herbal remedies for their livelihood. They purchased much of their meat and produce from their neighbors. The Duncans never begged. They always paid promptly for their purchases.

On this particular morning, Adam wanted to purchase a gallon of sorghum syrup, which Dad always made in very large quantities. Adam paid for the syrup and paused a moment at the door. "Ma'am," he said, "my madam and me would be mighty obliged if you would let your daughter come along with us on an herb hunt."

If I had submitted the same request, my mother would have treated it with a summary refusal. But asked by Adam, she appeared taken aback. "Well, I guess that … er, I … er, reckon so," she stammered.

"I 'spect we be going this coming Saturday," Adam announced. His mission accomplished, he left without another word.

As a general rule, Saturdays were special for me. It meant a trip to town after the morning chores were finished. And although money was scarce, there always seemed to be a dime or nickel leftover for a bag of gumdrops or peppermint sticks.

On this Saturday morning, however, my thoughts were not centered on town or candy counters. On my way to the Duncan house, I imagined myself preparing soothing potions and balms for healing the ills of mankind. Before the day was over, I would learn that, like any useful skill, herb lore is acquired by devoting hours of study and hard work.

I suppose in my naivete I expected to just go out into the woods and start picking herbs and roots like berries. I learned quickly that in herb gathering, one must have a close acquaintance with the mattock and spade. Another thing I learned was that Zora was not the acrimonious misanthrope she was reputed to be.

As we walked along, she explained some of the things she was interested in finding. "I want to be on the lookout for some boneset," she said. "It makes a lovely kettle of tea for healing fevers." "A lovely kettle of tea" was an expression I was to hear many times in the hours I spent with the Duncans.

Our first "strike" was a patch of sassafras. Sassafras tea, in addition to being a good tonic for colds and flu, is an excellent blood tonic and makes a delicious beverage. It can be mixed with carbonated water to make a tasty sarsaparilla. It was hard work digging the sweet, aromatic root, and soon my hands were very tired and sore.

In addition to various roots and plants, Adam took some bark from a wild cherry bush. "Cherry bark tea is good for chest colds," Zora explained. "It's also a good pep tonic. Makes you feel like yodeling." As I watched this big, rawboned woman work, I thought about how unjust people can be in judging someone harshly just because they happen to be a little eccentric.

At last, the Duncans finished their shopping in nature's big department store, and we were ready for the brewing phase of the operation.

Zora's kitchen was a far cry from kitchens in today's modern homes. It served as both dining room and kitchen. An old Warm Morning wood-burning stove sat within easy reach of a big, hand-hewn dining table which Adam had carved from oak as a wedding present for Zora. Zora had a number of iron kettles of assorted sizes which she used for boiling her water.

I watched carefully as Zora explained the process of making boneset tea. To one of the iron pots she added 1 teaspoon of powdered, dried petals of the boneset flower. Then she added 2 teaspoons of dried mint and 1 teaspoon of goldenseal root. After steeping the herbs in boiling water for 25 minutes, she strained the tea and sweetened it with honey.

Unlike many herbal practitioners, Zora did not add alcohol to her tonics. But it was not uncommon for people to lace their tonics liberally with whiskey or rum to give the temporary illusion of good feeling.

The day ended all too soon, and although I was tired, I enjoyed the feeling of accomplishment. It would not be my last visit to the Duncan home. Zora and I became good friends. She imparted much of her knowledge to me, and I spent many hours helping her and Adam gather roots and bark.

Alas, as all things end, so did my association with the Duncans. At Zora's death, Adam moved from the mountain, but not before making me a present of some of Zora's old teakettles. I still have the kettles, and they are a much-treasured part of my past. ◆

The Night We Ate The Onion Poultice

By Dale Morrison

This tastes just like good old onion poultice," I remarked. My hostess nearly had a stroke. But what I had said was sincere, and a great compliment; her onion flan was a culinary triumph.

My brother and I hit this planet during the first quarter of the century. It was a period of transition from Grandma's wisdom to medical science, and we were dosed liberally with both. There were no antibiotics as yet, and most drugs were suspect.

Our Grandma lived next-door, so we got the fringes of her benefits. We were made to drink boneset tea to "bring out the measles," and when we rebelled, Grandma told us we ought to be glad it wasn't sheep nanny tea, the remedy used for the same purpose during her childhood.

During Christmas vacation in 1925, little brother Al and I came down with congested chests. Our condition did not respond to massive anointings with mentholated salve, Mama's old standby. She rubbed our chests and backs with the menthol-and-pine mixture, poked it up our noses, made us swallow it in gooey lumps, and forced us to breathe in huge steamy drafts from a bowl of hot water afloat with salve, a towel draped over our head and the bowl. Had we known about allergic reactions back then, we would have manufactured one—and fast. To this day I can't stand menthol cough drops.

Then Mama and Grandma got into an argument about whether you were supposed to starve a cold and feed a fever, or feed a cold and starve a fever. They decided to play it safe and starve us, since we were running one degree of fever.

Consequently our next few meals were pitiful. Breakfast was one slice of dry toast and a cup of very weak tea. Lunch was toast and cambric tea, a Victorian disaster made by adding a half-cup of boiling water and a teaspoonful of sugar to a half-cup of skim milk. Ugh!

We had a little more for supper. (We were supposed to be grateful.) Supper was toast, a poached egg and cambric tea. When Brother suggested that Mama boil the tops of our overshoes if we were so poor, she gave him a dirty look.

We were allowed one indulgence—horehound sucks. These hard amber sticks of old-fashioned candy were to be broken into small chunks and allowed to dissolve on the tongue like lozenges. We promptly chewed them up and asked for more. Mama scolded us roundly, explaining that they were

We held a whispered consultation and then humbly asked to be allowed to creep downstairs to watch them make the poultices.

medicine, and medicine was not to be treated frivolously. As soon as Mama left the room we gobbled up the rest of the horehound sticks. Two hours later she spanked us.

We cried; we beat the wall; we howled "Food! Food!" like prisoners in a dungeon. It had no effect.

Mama said, "Quit your playacting. You're not starved yet. If you were really hungry, you'd know it."

That did it! We planned to climb out the window and sneak over to the store to buy cookies with our dime bank money, as there was no way to sneak anything from the kitchen. The stairway led to the dining room and the dining room led to the kitchen. There was no other path from our isolation, and Mama or Grandma was always there. At night our parents slept in the room between us and the stairs.

But "playacting" was the key word. We decided to act weak. We groaned realistically and flopped our arms listlessly when we finished our skimpy meals.

"So hungry," I would sob.

"Please," my brother would sob, "more!"

We laid it on thick. We pretended to be too feeble to feed ourselves. We let our voices sink to the merest whisper. We stared soulfully through our bangs at our captors.

Finally Grandma said, "This has gone on long enough."

Mama agreed. "The children need poultices on their chests."

Then they got into an argument about which kind of poultice it should be: bread poultice, flour-and-onion poultice, or mustard poultice?

Al and I clung to each other. Bread? Onions? Wasted on a poultice? Even the mustard sounded appetizing.

They compromised by making a bread-and-onion poultice with a touch of mustard. This was wonderful! Tantalized by the prospect, we held a whispered consultation and then humbly asked to be allowed to creep downstairs to watch them make the poultices.

Have you ever worn an old-fashioned, homemade poultice? Ours were really something. Grandma measured our chests and found clean cloth sugar sacks to match. Mama crumbled dry bread into a big pan as if she were making dressing. Over this she cut a huge mound of home-grown onions. She sprinkled on some ground mustard and tossed all the ingredients together. Then she stirred in enough boiling water to make a doughy mass. My brother and I got underfoot as much as possible during the process.

We watched carefully while Grandma spread the mixture inside the sugar sacks, then stitched the ends shut and sewed several monstrous tacks in each poultice to keep the contents from lumping together. Finally she sewed tapes at the four corners. Then Mama rushed us back upstairs and Grandma followed, carrying the soaking poultices in a basin of hot water.

The poultices were duly wrung out and slapped on our shrinking chests. The tapes were tied around our necks and waists. A clean old towel was folded over each poultice to protect our nightclothes which were buttoned snuggly up to our chins.

We tried to relax our quivering stomachs as the aroma of mustard and onions rose around us. The dear ladies covered us with blankets and comforts, turned the gas fire down to four inches, switched off the light and tiptoed away, whispering as though we were already snoring.

As soon as I heard the last stair tread creak below I was up on one elbow. "Did you get the stuff?" I hissed.

I could see my brother across the room in the flickering firelight as he rummaged under his pillow. "Right here," he grunted. "Both the salt and the pepper. What did you rescue?"

"Two spoons and a scissors," I chortled, tossing aside my covers and reaching for my fleece-lined bedroom slippers. The spoons were in the left toe, the scissors in the right. We hopped

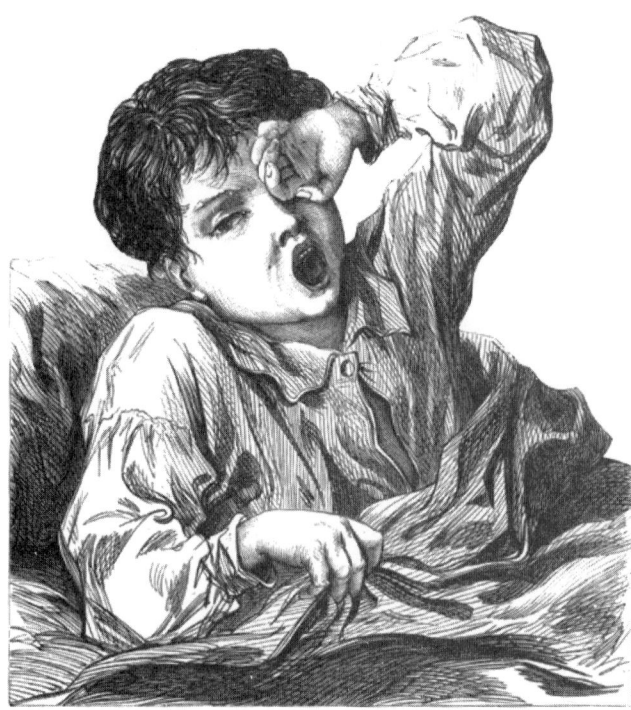

out of bed and hurried to the old brick hearth.

"Sorry, no plates," I said as I turned up the fire. While the flames rushed blue and gold up the hairy asbestos sheet, we divested ourselves of our poultices by cutting the tapes. We ripped out the tailor tacks and chopped into the sacks. The bread and onions were still hot and steaming. Using our towels for a tablecloth, we sat cross-legged on the floor and applied salt and pepper vigorously.

Nothing had ever tasted so good! The mustard gave our feast just the right edge. I believe we would have eaten every bite of it, even if it had been all flour and mustard!

We spooned every bit of that fragrant mess into our eager mouths. Yes, we even turned the sacks wrong side out and scraped. There was over a quart of the mixture in each sack. (Little kids in our family always *were* chesty.) Bulging full, we grinned at each other in the firelight.

"So how do we explain the empty sacks, Sister dear?" Al asked.

"We tell the truth, Brother love," said I. "After all, we probably won't have to explain anything until morning."

"They can't make us cough up our food then," he giggled.

We stretched our legs toward the flames and basked in silence for a bit, always with an ear tuned to the downstairs sounds. Then, when the

sixth sense children have told us it was time, we turned the fire back down and crept to our beds. "That was delicious," I said.

The last thing I heard was Al muttering, "Oh food, food, food … oh dreamy, dreamy mess."

We woke at dawn to smells of coffee and bacon drifting up the stairs. The first thing Al said was, "I'm hungry." He yawned, stretching, and then gasped, "I'm all well!"

I felt good, too. The wheeze and sniffles were gone; my chest was open and free. Every breath tingled with freshness all the way down. "Oh, whee!" I said. "Do you think they know?"

"We'll find out," Al muttered, making a box turtle of himself under the covers.

When Mama came up with her "happy morning face you put on for sick children to show them you care," we jumped out at her before she had time to ask, "And how do you feel?"

"We're well!" we shouted. "We're not a bit sick!"

"I can breathe!" Al said, popping the rubber buttons on his sleeper with a swelling demonstration.

"I can sing!" I cried, hopping up and down. "'High-ho, the dairy-oh, the farmer in the dell!'"

"My goodness," said Mama. "It was the onion poultice. Well, you had better take them off now."

"We can't," Al told her. "We ate them."

"Oh, p'shaw," Mama said. "It's time to take them off. They must be cold and clammy by now."

"Not on your nanny," squealed Al. "They're warm and safe."

"Inside us," I explained. "If you don't believe us, look." And I pointed to the two sad, stiff bags on the hearth.

"You have to be teasing," Mama said. "What did you do with the onions?"

"We told you—we ate them!" we cried.

"You can't have; people don't eat poultices, they wear them," she insisted. Then she looked at our chins. "Why did you do it?"

"Because we were hungry," I said.

"Because you starved us," Al added. "And I'm hungry again. We're not sick anymore. So we can eat bacon and eggs and oatmeal and bananas."

"Because we're well," I insisted.

"I don't know what your grandma will say," Mama sighed. "Get dressed and come downstairs."

We were deep in our second cups of cocoa when Grandma arrived. Our toast was covered with quince honey. We were polishing off a strictly normal breakfast at last with strictly normal appetites.

"Land sakes!" Grandma exclaimed, puffing in with a basket of eggs. "What's this?"

"The poultices worked," Mama said dryly, glaring at us.

"We ate them," Al squealed.

"They were good! They were glorious," I added.

Grandma began to laugh. After a bitter pause, Mama began to laugh too. They laughed until they had to wipe the tears from their eyes with the corners of their aprons.

After that, bread-and-onion pudding with a touch of mustard was known at our house as "The Children's Fabulous Cold and Fever Remedy." But it never again tasted quite as it did the night of the feast beside the firelight. The best batch came right out of the poultice bag. ◆

More Sound Advice From
The American Frugal Housewife

All herbs should be carefully kept from the air. Herb tea, to do any good, should be *very strong*.

Herbs should be gathered while in blossom. If left till they have gone to seed, the strength goes into the seeds. Those who have a little patch of ground will do well to raise the most important herbs; and those who have not, will do well to get them in quantities from some friend in the country; for apothecaries make very great profit upon them.

Sage is very useful, both as a medicine for headache—when made into tea—and for all kinds of stuffiness, when dried and rubbed into powder. It should be kept tight from the air.

Summer savory is excellent to season soup, broth and sausages. As a medicine, it relieves the colic.

Hyssop tea is good for sudden colds and disorders of the lungs. It is necessary to be very careful about exposure after taking it; it is peculiarly opening to the pores.

Motherwort tea is very quieting to the nerves. Students and people troubled with wakefulness find it useful.

Thoroughwort is excellent for dyspepsy and every disorder occasioned by indigestion. If the stomach be foul, it operates like a gentle emetic.

Catnip, particularly the blossoms, is good to prevent a threatened fever. It produces a fine perspiration. It should be taken in bed, and the patient kept warm.

Housekeepers should always dry leaves of the burdock and horseradish. Burdocks warmed in vinegar, with the hard, stalky parts cut out, are very soothing, applied to the feet; they produce a sweet and gentle perspiration. Horseradish is more powerful. It is excellent in cases of the ague, placed on the part affected, warmed in vinegar and clapped.

Few people know how to keep the flavor of sweet marjoram, the best of all herbs for broth and stuffing. It should be gathered in bud or blossom, and dried in a tin-kitchen at moderate distance from the fire; when dry, it should be immediately rubbed, sifted and corked up in a bottle carefully. ◆

SAGE

Medicinal Cures From The Country Kitchen

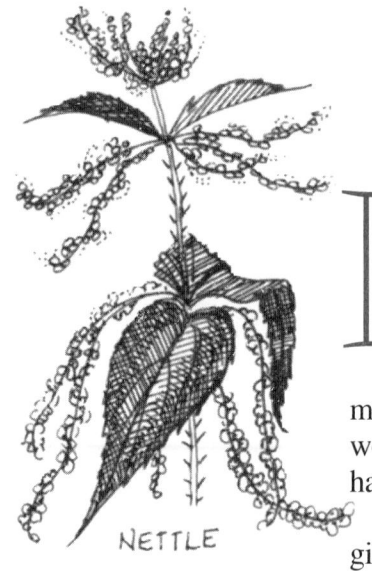

NETTLE

I n the good old days, people did not run to the doctor for every little ache or pain. Sometimes, they didn't go to the doctor for big aches or pains either. Doctoring cost money and money was often scarce.

Instead, people picked plants and herbs and concocted their own medicines right in the kitchen. Amazingly, some of the medicines worked quite well. Since the ingredients were all natural, they rarely had undesirable side effects.

The following material is not intended as medical advice but is given for information only.

Preparing Plant Parts for Home Use

Try to pick plants and leaves in the morning after the dew has dried but before the heat of the day. Essential oils are at their highest potency at this time.

Roots should be dug at the hottest point of the day. The heat drives the sap into the roots at that time.

Barks can be gathered at any time.

Take care when gathering plants and herbs in this present day that they have not been recently exposed to herbicides, pesticides or chemical fertilizers.

Blood-Purifying Tea

    4 parts dandelion root
    4 parts chicory root
    4 parts witch grass root
    1 part fennel seed

Mix ingredients together. Make a tea by boiling 1 or 2 tablespoons in water for 1 minute. Cool and strain. Dose: 2 tablespoons ½ hour after meals.

Migraine Headaches

    1 ounce St. Johnswort
    1 ounce primrose flowers
    1 ounce blessed thistle
    1 ounce lavender flowers

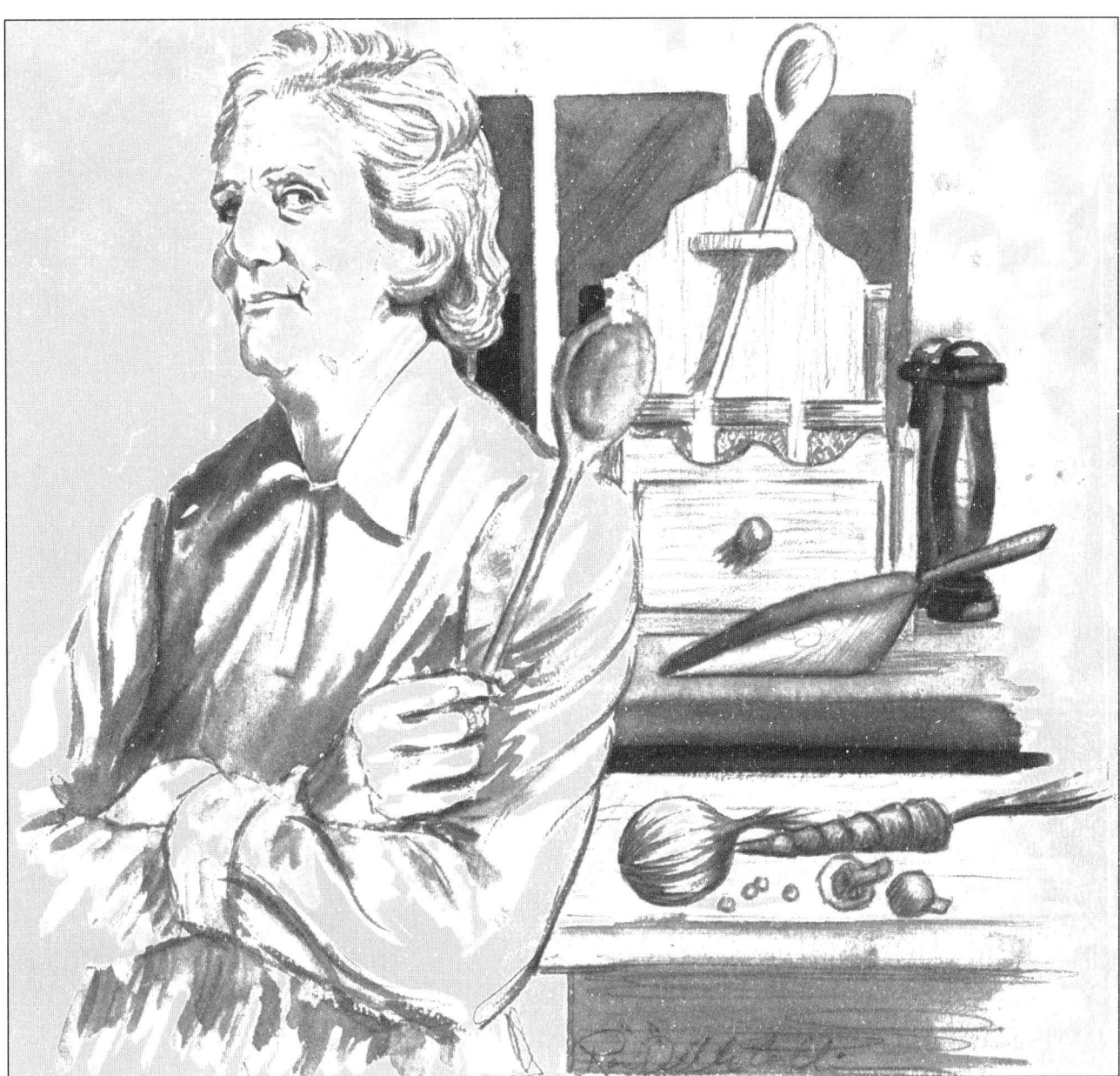

1 ounce sweet balm leaves
2 ounces peppermint leaves
3 ounces valerie root

Mix ingredients together; then take 1 or 2 heaping teaspoons and mix with boiling water. Drink 3 cups every day.

For Whooping Cough

Take chestnut leaves and boil them until the water is red. Add sufficient sugar and boil down to a thin syrup. Give the patient a tablespoonful when coughing.

Cure for Poisoning

Pour boiling water over a few mayapples. Cool; take ½ teaspoon every 10–15 minutes until relieved.

Cure for Neuralgia

Make a tea from bull-nettle leaves and drink. Lay a poultice of the leaves on the affected parts.

For Boils

Make a tea from sycamore bark. Drink instead of water. It's a sure cure.

For Dropsy

Fill a quart jar half-full of rosemary leaves. Pour over this sufficient wine to fill the jar. Let stand 24 hours. Take 2–4 tablespoons morning and night.

For Bleeding Piles
Take 2 large handfuls of peach tree leaves and fry them in 2 tablespoons of lard until the leaves are black and the lard is dark. Strain and let cool. Apply as you would any other salve.

For Infected Eyes
Make a tea from the pith of the sassafras tree and bathe eyes. Do not use the bark.

Bull-Nettle Cough Syrup
Take a large handful of dried roots of bull nettle and add to 1 quart of water. Boil down until only 1 pint remains. Add enough sugar to make a syrup.

For Poison Ivy
Rub goldenrod leaves in cold water. Wash affected parts with this whenever it itches.

For Teething Babies
Boil a small handful of ground ivy with a small handful of blackberry root. Strain and sweeten. Give to teething babies for relief of diarrhea.

Cancer Cure
Make and drink tea made from red clover.

For Anemia
Gather leaves of the black walnut tree while they are green. Dry them and make a strong tea, but not in an aluminum kettle. Drink instead of water.

For Worms
Make a strong infusion of the seed of the Jerusalem oak. Dose: 1 teaspoon mixed with sugar 3 times a day.

Asthma Relief
   3 parts coughwort
   3 parts plantain
   3 parts sage
   1 part silver mullein
Grind dried leaves together and add 2–4

heaping teaspoons to boiling water. Let cool 15 minutes, strain, and add 2 tablespoons honey.

For Bladder Infections
Use equal parts of:
   Linden flowers
   Elder flowers
   St. Johnswort
   German chamomile flowers
   Blackberry leaves
Grind dried leaves into powder and make into a tea. Drink three times a day.

For Dysentery
Make a tea from nettle leaves.

Plants Containing Iron
   Yellow dock
   Strawberry leaves
   Stinging nettles
   Silver weed
   Rest harrow
   Burdock
   Mullein leaves

Plants Containing Calcium
   Horsetail grass
   Toad flax
   Cleavers
   Shepherd's purse
   Mistletoe
   Chamomile
   Dandelion

Plants Containing Potassium
   Walnut leaves
   Mistletoe
   German chamomile flowers
   Plantain leaves
   Summer savory
   Birch bark
   Nettle leaves
   Borage
   Yarrow
   Mullein
   Oak bark
   Carrot leaves ◆

How to Cure a Cold

By Arlene Shovald

Even with all of today's medicines and knowledge, they still haven't found a cure for the common cold. Today, just as when Grandma was a girl, a cold has to run its course. The remedies available may make the patient more comfortable, but they don't cure him. And though modern methods of treating cold symptoms are undoubtedly easier to take, there is still some doubt as to whether they work any better than the old-fashioned ones.

Garlic was highly recommended as both cold preventative and cure. Italian youngsters wore small bags of garlic around their necks to ward off germs.

Onions, too, were supposed to fight off colds. A thoroughly obnoxious—but nevertheless effective—cough syrup was made in the hot oven of the old wood-burning cookstove by baking onions in plenty of sugar. The resulting syrup soothed coughs.

One little grandmother who had been a nurse during the Civil War tied asafetida gum in a little pouch and hung it from a string around her patient's neck. Asafetida is an Oriental plant of the carrot family, and a none-too-fragrant member at that!

I suspect that these old-fashioned methods worked, but not because they were medically appropriate treatments. They just smelled so bad that no one wanted to get close enough to spread any germs!

In the old days, preparing the goose for Christmas dinner left the cook with more than just a fine bird for roasting. The goose grease was saved and put away to treat colds throughout the year. Not only was it a fine chest rub, but a bit of it melted and given by the spoonful was good for a cold. If the cold hadn't made you sick enough, a spoonful of goose grease would finish the job!

Sweating seems to be frowned upon in modern society, but in the old days a good sweat—sometimes called a "stew"—was good for what ailed you when "what ailed you" was a cold. The patient went to bed with hot bricks at his feet and snuggled under a pile of comforters. Then he drank plenty of hot tea for the next hour or two until he'd worked up a good, dripping perspiration and literally "sweated it out." Those of Russian ancestry recommended that the tea be brewed from elder flowers and sweetened with honey.

In the North Woods, resin from the pine tree was used to treat colds. In the lumber camps, that hearty breed of timbermen noted for their health and gusto mixed pine pitch with hot water and honey to make a thick syrup for colds. They also inhaled steam from melted resin to heal inflammation and promote sound sleep.

By far the tastiest and most pleasant of the old remedies was the one my Grandma prescribed—hot lemonade, accompanied by a chest rub with camphorated oil. The lemonade tasted good and warmed the insides, and the camphor made the bedding smell all warm and cozy and induced sound, peaceful sleep—also important when treating a cold.

PEPPERMINT

Each nationality had its own preferred remedy back in those days when the United States was a big melting pot of nations. French mamas tied woolen stockings around their children's throats, "bundled" them, and sent them off to straw ticks or feather beds. But there was one stipulation: the sock must have been worn! Needless to say, a stuffed nose sometimes worked to the patient's advantage!

People don't have time for "bundling" any more and nobody wants to smell of garlic or onion syrup or, for that matter, old socks. Today the shelves in drugstores and supermarkets are loaded with modern aids for cold sufferers. Whether they do a better job is a matter of opinion; to each his own. But none can be more lovingly applied than the mustard plasters and goose grease that was tenderly slathered on little patients' chests by the gentle hands of old. ◆

Boil Up the Birch Bark

By Callie B. Young

In the days before prescription medicines were readily available, people like my grandparents used imagination and ingenuity to help relieve ailments and misery. Today we think of these remedies as "folk remedies," but at the time they defined a cultural system designed to cure or alleviate chronic health problems. Bark and roots were often used, and these folk remedies were passed from one generation to another.

These ingredients were kept on hand and were used to treat colds, fever, indigestion, sore throats, headaches, lesions and general aches and pains. The remedies were often given in the form of teas, syrups or salves. I remember some of the remedies my parents used; they were handed down from my paternal grandmother, and were made from the bark of the birch tree. My parents and grandparents believed this bark had medicinal qualities, and they made use of it.

Today the birch tree is often associated with spacious lawns and pastures, yielding its beauty and shade to man and animals. But in the days when medical relief depended in part on home remedies, the bark from the birch tree was more important than its shade and beauty.

We had a birch tree in our pasture near the barn. My dad would peel the bark from the tree with his pocketknife, letting the strippings drop into a lard bucket or other utensil from the kitchen cabinet.

My mother would wash the bark, then put it in a pot, stoke the wood stove, and slowly bring this concoction to a boil. When the mixture was a murky brown, she strained it through a cloth sugar sack. After she poured it into a crock, she covered it with a flour sack. Later she would divide it into three portions. Different ingredients were added to each to make various remedies.

To a quart of the mixture, my mother added ½ cup of sugar, 1 tablespoon of honey, and 6 sage leaves. After heating it, she added a level teaspoon of alum. When the blend cooled, my mother poured her "birch-bark tea," as she called it, into a half-gallon fruit jar with a zinc lid. We children were given small doses of the tea for coughs, bad colds and sore throats.

Spring was tonic time at our house. The birch-bark tea was the cure for the dread disease we youngsters had each spring, when our mother said we were "bilious." She believed this tea not only eliminated biliousness, but also purified the blood, and even cured a stomach-ache. (I learned years later that biliousness was caused by a sluggish liver secretion which caused one to be cross or bad-tempered, and was not a dread disease at all.)

For chest congestion, fever or croup, my mother made a thick syrup from some of the birch-bark mixture. In a long-handled stewer she poured a large portion of the liquid from the crock, added 2 tablespoons of honey, 1 of lard, and to thicken it, another of flour. This was slowly cooked until it had a thick, syrupy texture. It was then given, a spoonful at a time, to her ailing children. The sweet, syrupy mixture soothed many a fevered brow and brought relief from an irritating cough on a cold winter night.

The remaining mixture in the crock was made into a salve. Cornmeal, mutton tallow (made with the fat from sheep) mixed with alum, salt, lard and a sprinkling of ground cloves were mixed with the liquid and poured into a black skillet. This was cooked—stirred continuously to keep it from sticking—until it became a thick salve. Stored in a covered container, it was used for a variety of injuries and ailments.

Rubbed on the chest and covered with flannel, this clove-scented salve relieved some chest congestion and helped cuts and sores. The afflicted area could be bathed in warm, salty water; then the salve was applied and covered with a bandage.

Today the birch tree is often associated with spacious lawns and pastures, yielding its beauty and shade to man and animals. In the days when medical relief depended in part on home remedies, the bark from the birch tree was more important than its shade and beauty.

This salve would also relieve earache pain when rubbed into the ear. And, my mother rubbed this salve onto a flannel bib and put it around my little brother's neck when he had the croup.

Today penicillin and other miracle drugs are easily available. If we would take the time to read the list of ingredients used in the medicines dispensed by modern pharmacists, we would find that many of these drugs had their roots in folk medicine.

Most medicine cabinets today are well-stocked with cures for all ailments from toe itch to asthma attacks. If you should find your aspirin bottle empty and need a quick headache cure, then "boil up the birch bark" and make a pot of tea. When you drink it you may be in for a surprise. ◆

Herb Cures For Nervous Ills

By Elizabeth Hillman

Nowadays, anyone suffering from mental distress has tranquilizers or psychiatrists to help them, but our ancestors had other ideas! Shyness was treated with aromatic tea, to which 20 drops of a mixture of angelica and rum were added (perhaps the herb wasn't too important in that), or a less exciting dose of clover tea.

Nervous headaches were treated by "snorting" powdered basil leaves or by wearing a quilted cap stuffed with lavender flowers to bed. (The cap had to be made of red silk to be effective, though.) An American herbalist in 1940 had another recommendation for nervous headache—sprinkling vinegar and black pepper on brown paper and applying it to the forehead for relief. And we all thought the *Jack and Jill* nursery rhyme was just nonsense!

Depression was treated with white wine and sage or claret in which were steeped leaves of sage, hyssop, thyme, mint and marjoram.

If you were made uneasy by suspecting that the evil eye had been put on your house, you simply planted lemon trees, rosemary bushes, rue or artemisia in your garden, hung garlic in the house, and chewed cumin seeds.

A delightful tea was brewed to help "disturbances of the nerves"—equal parts of hops, clover, violets, lime flowers, orange peel, bee balm and valerian were mixed and stored, then one teaspoonful of the mixture was added to a cup of boiling water, steeped for five minutes, then filtered. Drunk three times a day, it was especially for neurasthenia.

Insomnia was helped with lettuce tea, chamomile with orange peel tea or poppy and

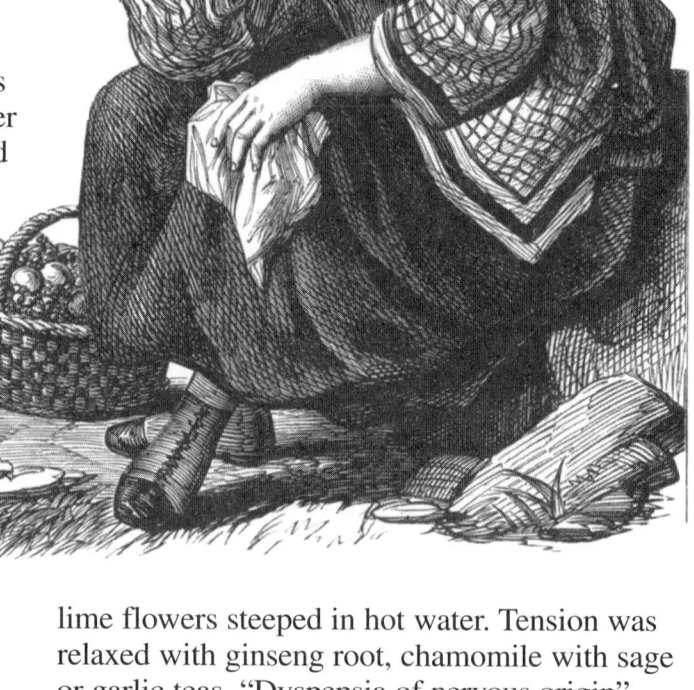

lime flowers steeped in hot water. Tension was relaxed with ginseng root, chamomile with sage or garlic teas. "Dyspepsia of nervous origin" was helped with anise tea.

Whether these cures actually work or not, an ancient idea still worth considering is that nervous ills can be helped with pleasant aroma. Remember the Victorian ladies and their vinaigrettes? The next time you feel low or tense, find a bottle of your favorite cologne (most contain aromatic herbs). Then lean back, close your eyes, sniff in the perfume and relax. ◆

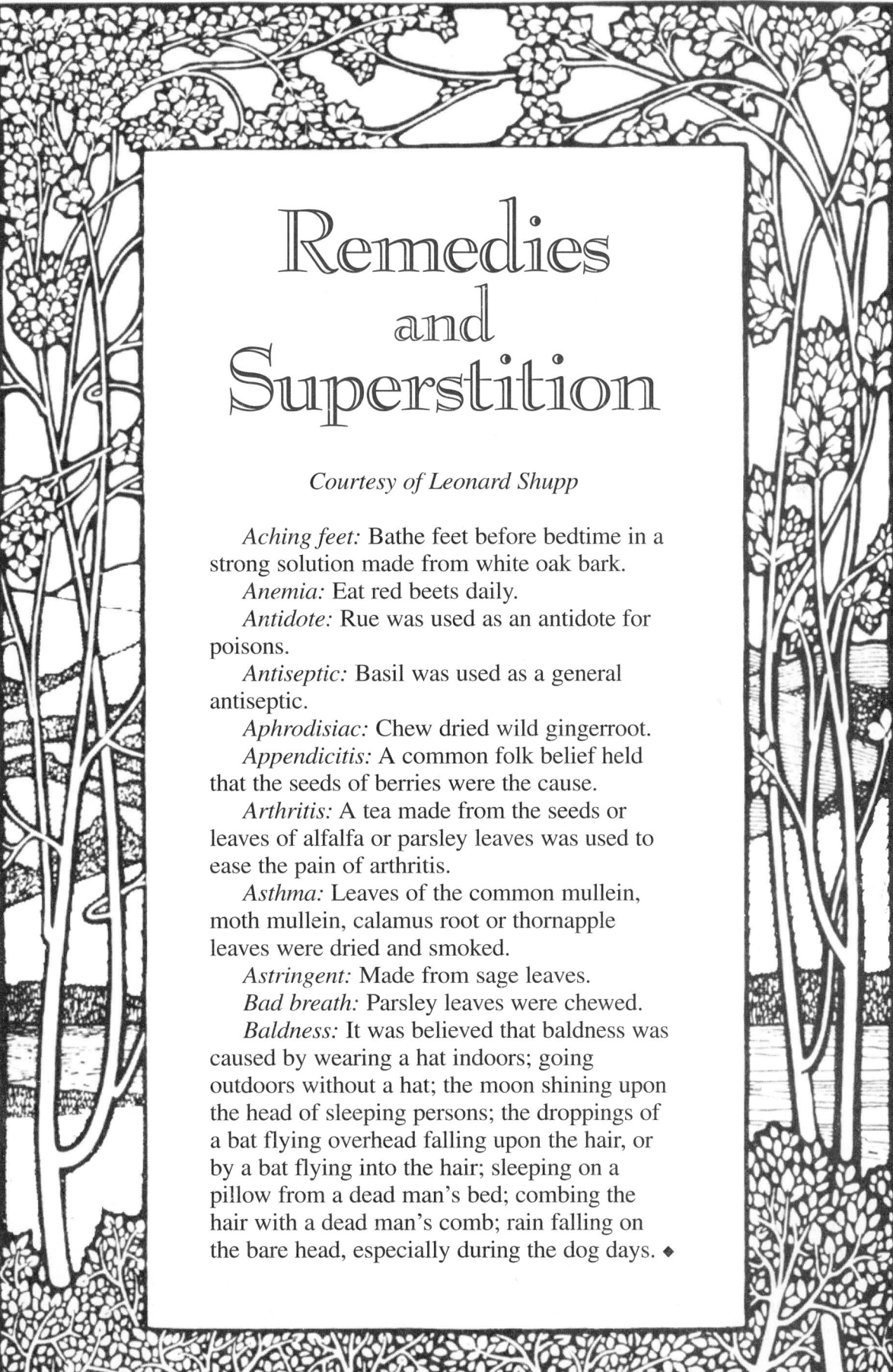

Remedies and Superstition

Courtesy of Leonard Shupp

Aching feet: Bathe feet before bedtime in a strong solution made from white oak bark.

Anemia: Eat red beets daily.

Antidote: Rue was used as an antidote for poisons.

Antiseptic: Basil was used as a general antiseptic.

Aphrodisiac: Chew dried wild gingerroot.

Appendicitis: A common folk belief held that the seeds of berries were the cause.

Arthritis: A tea made from the seeds or leaves of alfalfa or parsley leaves was used to ease the pain of arthritis.

Asthma: Leaves of the common mullein, moth mullein, calamus root or thornapple leaves were dried and smoked.

Astringent: Made from sage leaves.

Bad breath: Parsley leaves were chewed.

Baldness: It was believed that baldness was caused by wearing a hat indoors; going outdoors without a hat; the moon shining upon the head of sleeping persons; the droppings of a bat flying overhead falling upon the hair, or by a bat flying into the hair; sleeping on a pillow from a dead man's bed; combing the hair with a dead man's comb; rain falling on the bare head, especially during the dog days. ◆

Tansy Cures And Recipes

By Gladys Reed Robinson

One of the most beneficial plants I know of in the herb garden is the herb *Tanacetum vulgare.* Not only was it found in the herb gardens just outside the kitchen doors in the good old days; but country roadsides and creek banks were decked out with it wearing its beautiful dress of yellow during the summer months.

The blossoms consist of dense corymbs of numerous small, rich yellow heads which begin to appear in August and continue until the first frost. The upright unbranched stems rise 2 to 3 feet, and bear divided, deeply cut compound leaves. The strong, peculiar odor is much diminished by drying.

Its sister plant, *Tanacetum crispum,* has similar flowers but a much lacier, fuller leaf formation which is much better for harvesting since you will not have to harvest such a large amount to yield a generous quantity of dried tansy.

Tansy may be cut back in late summer, washed thoroughly to remove soil or insect particles, and then hung up to dry in a shed, barn or room away from direct sunlight and dampness. When the leaves feel crisp to the touch, they may be stripped from the stems, placed on a board and crushed to the desired texture with a rolling pin. Then they should be stored in an airtight container. Some of the seeds may be saved to sprinkle on cookies instead of sugar

Tansy will survive in most any soil except damp or wet places.

The ancients used tansy to preserve meat and repel flies. Tansy leaves placed on pantry shelves will rid them of ants. Leafy tips of tansy are used in cosmetic ointment and in the liqueur Chartreuse. Tansies, a kind of cookie, were made in England as far back as the 17th century, and were given to the poor at Easter in honor of the paschal feast.

If your garden is infested with large anthills, clusters of tansy roots placed directly in the center of the hill will do away with the ants. I speak of this from personal experience.

Tea made from dried tansy, chilled and served with a little lemon, makes a very pleasant and conversational thirst quencher. It may even be mixed with another favorite variety of tea. I remember my grandmother saying that a jar of chilled tansy tea always accompanied

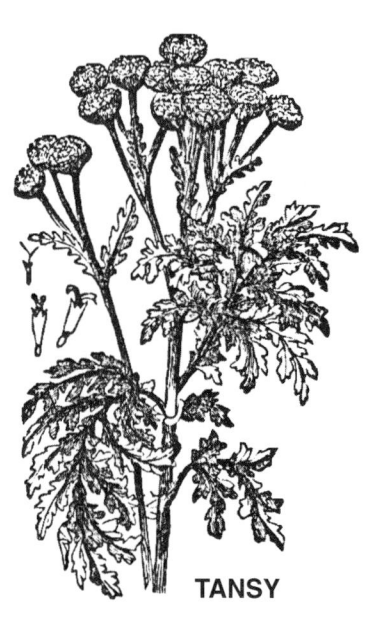

TANSY

the men to the fields. This was long before the days of mechanical devices, and when the men and horses left for the fields, they usually did not return until the end of the day.

Dried tansy may also be sewn into little sachets to be placed in the clothes closet or bureau drawers. Equal parts of crushed tansy and ground cloves make an excellent combination and sell very well at church fairs.

I have experimented with the herb and have published my own recipes for tansy cookies and biscuits. I usually serve the bread as a novelty item at parties or for afternoon tea. Cookies and biscuits may be used likewise.

From its bright yellow flowers which make lovely dried arrangements to its aromatic leaves which repel insects, tansy is a valuable old-time herb.

Tansy Bread

2 cups boiling water or boiling potato water
1 cup rolled oats
1 tablespoon butter
½ cup brown sugar
1 dry yeast cake dissolved in ½ cup warm water
1 teaspoon salt
1 teaspoon nutmeg
1 teaspoon celery seed
2 tablespoons parsley flakes
1 pimiento, chopped fine
1 teaspoon Bell's Seasoning
1½ tablespoons crumbled, dried tansy
2 heaping tablsepoons grated cheese (optional)
4½ cups sifted flour

Pour boiling water over rolled oats. Add butter and brown sugar and set aside for 2 hours.

Then add dissolved yeast, salt, nutmeg, celery seed, parsley flakes, chopped pimiento, Bell's seasoning, tansy, and cheese, if desired. Add flour.

Mix well and allow to stand until it is light, then stir down; divide into loaves or rolls. Put in buttered tins and allow to rise again. When double in bulk, brush with melted butter and bake in hot oven (375–400 degrees) for 20 minutes. Reduce heat to 350 degrees and bake until done, depending upon size of loaves.

I like to use potato water, as I think it helps keep the bread fresh longer, and the cheese, too, has a tendency to help keep it fresh as well as adding to the flavor. This bread is delicious toasted and goes well with cold meats and potato salad.

A patch of tansy planted here and there in your flower garden will give you many years of use, pleasure and enjoyment.

Tansy Tea Biscuits

1 cup scalded milk
¼ cup butter
2 tablespoons sugar
½ yeast cake dissolved in warm water
1 egg, well beaten
2 cups bread flour
1½ teaspoons crumbled, dried tansy

Mix all ingredients well. Let rise, then spoon into gem pans. Let rise again and carefully place in oven. Bake at 375–400 degrees about 20 minutes. Serve hot.

Tansy Cookies

2½ cups sifted flour
1 teaspoon baking powder
½ teaspoon soda
½ teaspoon salt
½ cup shortening or butter (softened)
1 cup sugar
2 eggs, unbeaten
1 teaspoon vanilla (optional)
1½ teaspoons crumbled, dried tansy
1 tablespoon milk

Sift together flour, baking powder, baking soda and salt into a large bowl. Add remaining ingredients.

Beat until well-blended, about 3 minutes with a mixer. Roll out to ⅛-inch thickness on a lightly floured board. Cut with cookie cutter which has been dipped in flour. Bake about 10 minutes in 400-degree oven, or until golden brown. Makes about 2½ dozen large, crisp cookies.◆

A Second Opinion

By Norma Stirm

Too bad that Gramma's favorite girl
Has finally had to go
Where doctors send sick children,
But what do doctors know?
I could have cured you right at home,
With senna tea and spice.
But NO! Your modern mother
Wouldn't hear to my advice!
I have these ancient remedies,
All family-tried and true.
But do you think she'd let me try
Them out, dear child, on you?
My mother always cured my cold,
When I first made a fuss,
With hot fried onions 'round my neck
To clear my sinuses!
But NO! Your mother gave a yell
And darned near hit the sky!
The thought of steaming onions
Just started her to cry.

Then I remembered goose grease!
Rubbed into each armpit,
T'would open up your pores and let
Your fever out a bit.
I told her of a gargle
That always worked first-rate—
Rainwater mixed with lavender
And ammonia carbonate.
Although I pleaded, she refused
My mustard plaster cure.
If Grandpa were alive today,
He'd prove that it was sure!
I offered her some skunk oil
To rub upon your chest.
In no uncertain terms, she scorned
This offer, with the rest.
I only pray, dear Jenny,
That the doctors there come through
With help enough to get you *home*
So *I* can take care of you!

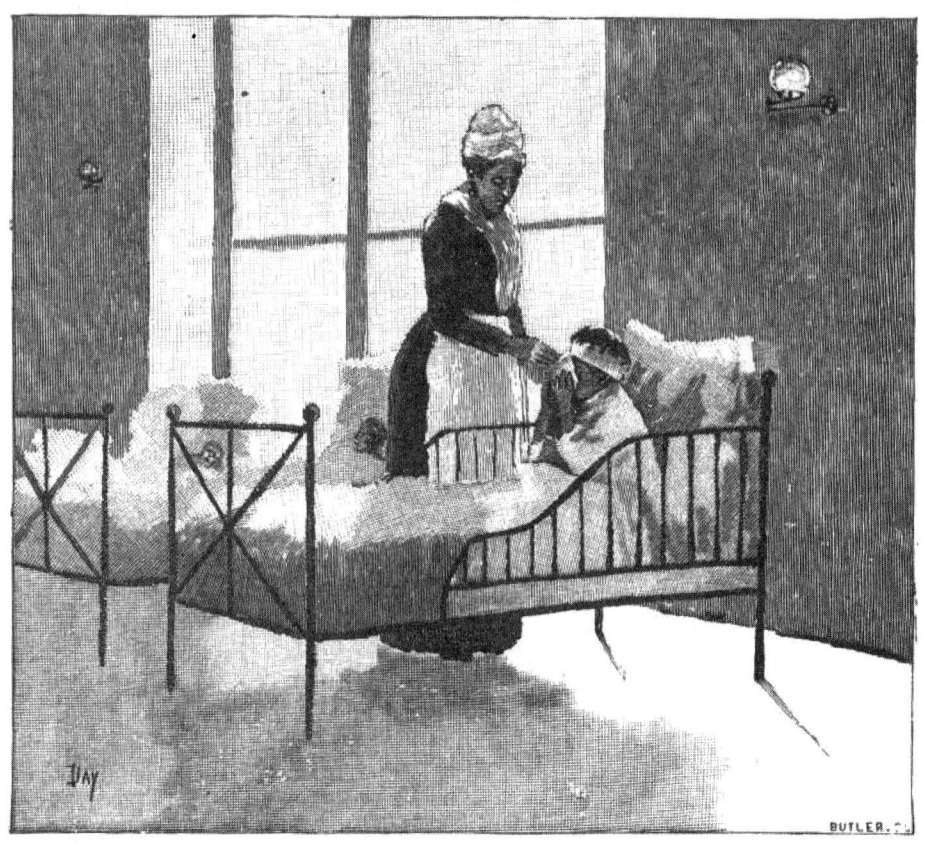

Home Remedies

Poison Ivy

Years ago, my brother and I played in marshes near our home where we got poison ivy on our feet and hands. At night when we couldn't rest, Father would get up and pick plantain leaves, chop these up and apply it on our blisters.

There probably isn't a remedy for poison ivy I haven't tried, but two work better than all the rest. One is to apply tobacco juice. If this idea seems too revolting, try remedy number two. Get water from the pail in which a blacksmith dips horseshoes. Be sure the water is not fresh but has been in use for some time. Apply freely and soon the itching will abate.

Esther Cornish, Gillette, N.J.

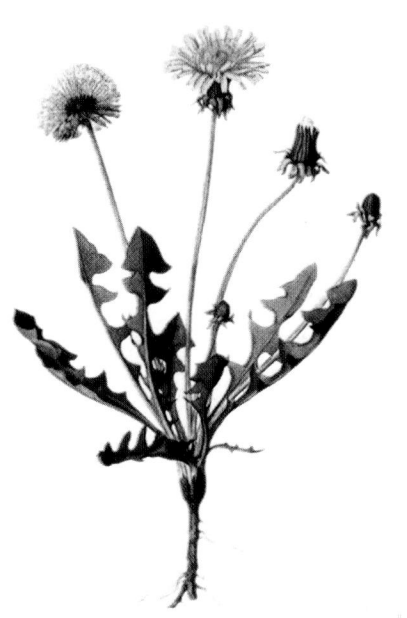

Tonics

Mama used to give us spring tonics. First was sassafras tea. It was to cure us of whatever winter illness might still be ailing us. We would say, "But Mama, we don't like it!"

She would answer, "So drink it anyhow; it's good for you!" We would drink it and not talk back.

Next came dandelion greens. The first leaf that appeared would set Mama out gathering them by the bucketful. She cooked them, and again we protested. Again she said, "So eat them; they're good for you." To this day, the first warm day of spring finds me looking for the first dandelions.

To cook delicious dandelion greens, gather a large amount of greens, at least a full peck sack, as they cook down so much. Look them over carefully, using only the largest leaves. Wash carefully. Cook in a kettle of water with a pinch of soda. Drain; repeat. Then cook until tender in a lightly salted water and drain. Brown a few bread cubes in hot fat. Add greens. Cook until well-blended. May be served with butter or vinegar.

Elnora Harris, Atchison, Kan.

Cough Syrup

This recipe for cough syrup has been in my family for years. I know it's at least 95 years old and maybe older. It originated in Missouri.

Mix together:
⅓ cup honey
½ teaspoon cream of tartar
1 teaspoon flower of sulphur
Take ⅛ teaspoon as often as every 1½ hours, as needed.

Mary Chatman, Yakima, Wash.

Home Cures

For a sore throat, put skunk oil on a rag around the neck.

For an earache, apply sweet oil on cotton and insert in ear.

To break up a cold, make a sack of rags, heat it and put it on your chest. Put a towel over it.

For a cold, drink hot sage tea. Raise your own sage on a bush. In the fall, cut the leaves and lay out on paper to dry. When dry, pour boiling water over it.

For a puncture wound or sore, make a hot bread-and-milk poultice.

For colds and sore throats, chop onions finely; put them in a saucer on the back of the cookstove. When the juice comes out, drink it.

Residents of Evangelical Free Church Home
Boone, Iowa

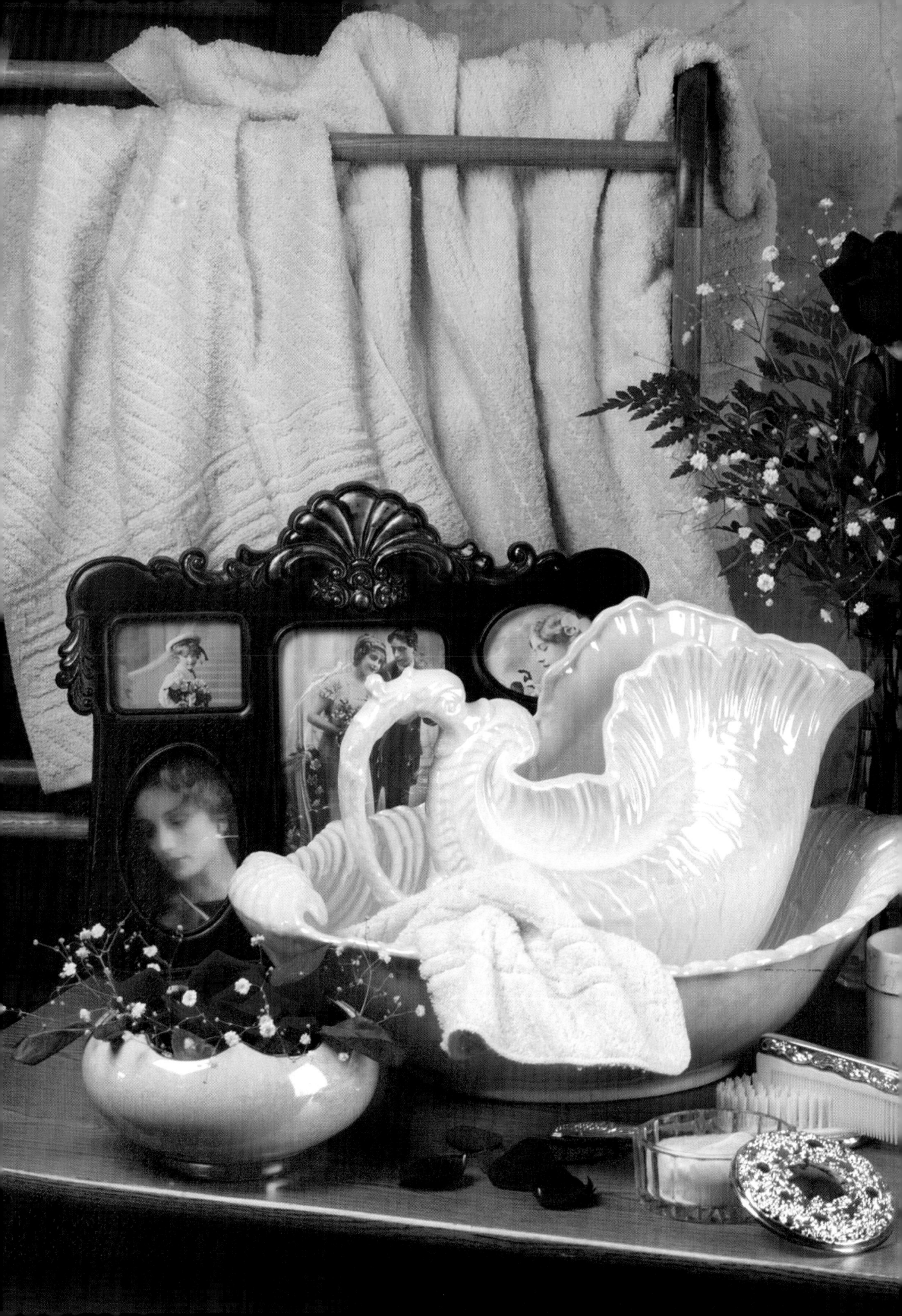

Chapter 2

MOTHER'S AND OTHERS' REMEDIES

Daddy was a healer—of that there was no doubt. He knew how to heal a hurt puppy's leg. He knew how to heal Mama's periodic hurt feelings. And he knew how to heal an ornery little boy's ills, both imagined and real.

He could heal a bout of "school fever"—you know, the mysterious malady that strikes otherwise healthy youngsters on a beautiful spring morning just before schooltime. He healed it with the promise of a day of chores to "work the fever out."

He could heal a "crick" in my neck with a short period of massage followed by a quick snap of my head that would either run the crick out or break my neck trying.

One of my fondest memories of Daddy, however, is that of him gently blowing smoke from his pipe into my ear whenever I had an earache. It showed me that this strong, barrel-chested man could also have the character of compassion and gentleness. As I read these stories of such mothers and other healers, I am reminded of Daddy and his natural capacity to love—and to heal. Enjoy and remember those best of times!

—Ken Tate

Crooked Finger's Natural Healing

By Trula Johnson

Editor's Note: I first met Trula Johnson several years ago after she had submitted a story of her life with her grandmother for publication in Good Old Days. *My great-grandmother was likewise a Native American, a Cherokee, so Trula and I spent a great deal of time talking of our roots. Many of the sachem's remedies were passed along to the white man and came to be part of our earlier days' customs and traditions. I felt it was fitting to have this memory of Crooked Finger in this book of home remedies.*

My grandmother, Crooked Finger, was a Native American—a member of the Delaware tribe—born in Joplin, Mo., in 1871. She learned to practice natural healing with herbs long before she met and married Jim Turney, who brought her to Oklahoma Territory in 1888.

In 1937, I was 9 years old and living at Fort Cobb, Okla. It was a cool morning in late September, and I was fighting off a cold.

"A wild Indian who won't follow my advice!" was Grandma's favorite description of me. I was a skinny, rebellious girl who often lived with Grandma when my divorced mother couldn't make ends meet.

> *"It embarrassed me for her to speak of my prophecies. I want to be remembered for using natural healing herbs."*

"Good health is the result of natural, healthful living in mind and body," Grandma often said. She was a firm believer in Genesis 1:29: "And God said, Behold, I have given you every herb bearing seed, which is upon the face of all the earth, and every tree in which is the fruit of a tree yielding seed; to you it shall be for meat."

Smiling her special doctor's smile, Grandma nodded her still-lovely head which was framed by straight raven hair. Her honey-colored skin glowed with radiant health even though she was 66.

"Sabbeleu," she called me by my childhood name that means *shining water reflection*, "you must eat this special chicken soup spiced with garlic, chili peppers and horseradish to loosen that thick bunch of crud in your nose and chest."

"But it doesn't taste good like your usual soup does," I protested.

"Medicine isn't supposed to taste good. Finish it up now, and drink

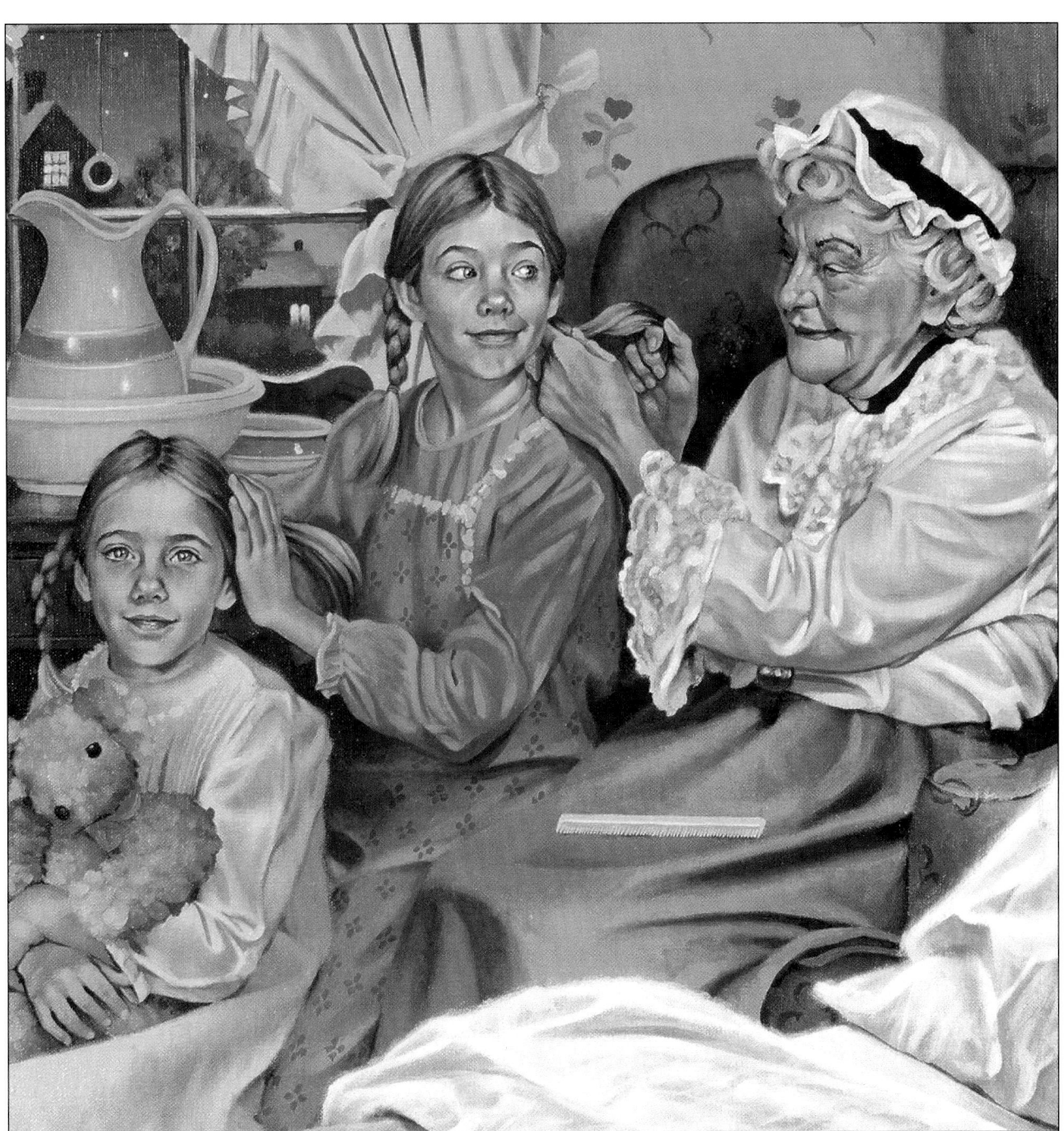

your herb tea made with anise and sage. You want to get well so you can go back to school, don't you?"

"Yes … but tell me a story about your recent sachem visit to heal one of your sick ones."

She sat down beside me at the old wooden table in the old farmhouse and smiled as she began her story:

Running Wolf, Gathers Flowers' husband, came

to me just a few days ago to help him with his sick wife's strange illness.

"Crooked Finger, honored sachem healer, my wife is in bed and the white doctor, called Dr. Luke, is unable to heal or make her feel better with his pills and tonics," he said.

"Tell me her miseries so I'll know what herbs to take with me when we go to your tent," I said.

"She complains of evil spirits in her arms,

fingers and legs," Running Wolf said. "And when she walks, she limps and moans."

I gathered my herb jars, carefully saved by those who could afford to buy them, noting the neat labels which named what herb each jar contained. Then I accepted his outstretched fingers and climbed onto the frisky horse. We were soon galloping toward his tent a few miles away.

When we arrived we dismounted and he led me into his home. Gathers Flowers was on a small platform bed, and she tried to smile as I approached her.

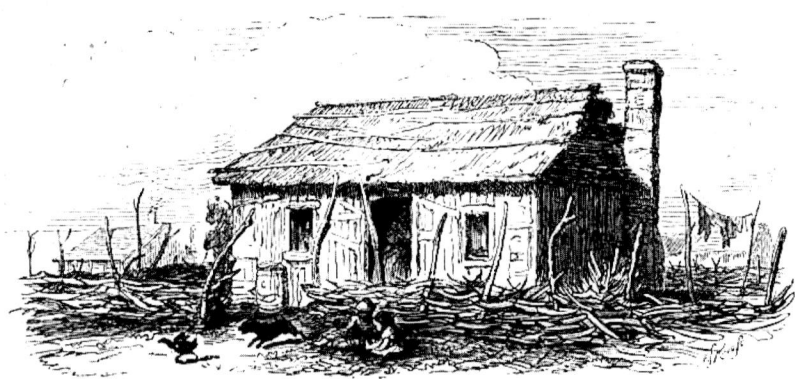

"I came as soon as your husband told me of your sickness," I said. "Running Wolf, leave us now. I need to talk to Gathers Flowers alone."

He glanced at his wife, his concern reflected in his nutmeg-colored eyes. He left without another word.

I squatted down and looked into her eyes. I saw the white iris rim that reflected one of her complaints. I uncovered her and stared at her feet which were swollen, especially her big toe. With some thoughts forming in my mind, I began with some of my important questions.

"Tell me what hurts most," I instructed. "Your eyes show that you are not well, as well as your swollen feet."

"Pain begins in my small finger." She held up her left finger. "And it travels around until it hits my shoulders. My legs and arms cramp at night, but even when I walk, I hurt."

"Can you *edau* (empty your bowels) regularly? What do you eat?" I asked.

"No, I can't edau every day," she said, "and before this pain, I wheezed a lot—seemed to be hard to breathe. I know I don't eat right; I use the trading post's food too much...."

"You have what the salt (white) people call 'arthritis,'" I told her. "We call it 'evil spirits in the bones.' I'll leave you some herb tea, but you must quit smoking your corncob pipe, quit drinking firewater (alcohol), wear your moccasins, not white man's shoes, and soak your feet in hot and then cold water each day. Eat cottage cheese; you know how to make it, and you don't like milk, I know.

"Eat more fish," I continued, "not so much red meat as you do now. Rub your toes, tops and bottoms, for 30 minutes gently with stiff fingers, then rub your heels and bottoms and tops of your feet. Do the same to your hands. Have your husband use acupressure and walk. Enjoy the sunshine, even though it hurts to do so."

Finally I instructed her, "Quit worrying so much. Get involved with both whites and others. If you'll do this, you'll feel much better in a month or two. Will you do this for yourself?"

"Yes," she told me. "I don't want to hurt so much."

"I'll show you how to bunch your fingers for using acupressure and the spots to rub deeply," I promised, "and I'll give you the herbs for healing. Follow my advice for food and quit smoking your pipe and drinking too much alcohol. Get along with people better. Soon, you'll see a difference."

"You are a gifted healer, Crooked Finger," Gathers Flowers said. "I've also heard of your prophecies which almost always come true."

"Sabbeleu," Grandma said to me, "it embarrassed me for her to speak of my prophecies. I want to be remembered for using natural healing herbs."

Crooked Finger died in 1943, but she left her natural healing methods, her prophecies and the story of her life with me.

Many legends and myths were also her legacy, which I now like to share with my own grandchildren and others who enjoy hearing of the good old days. ◆

Grandma's Home Remedies

Some 60 years ago, I was at my grandmother's when I cut my finger very badly; it was bleeding freely. My grandmother's cook ran out onto the back porch and brought back a spiderweb. She placed it around the cut to stop the bleeding. It really worked.

My older sister said our mother's cook stopped the bleeding from a cut on her foot by smearing soot from the coal- and wood-burning stove on the cut. This also worked.

—**Christine Hawes**

When I was a child my mother had a cure for the stomachache which no child refused. In fact, my brother and I often "had the stomachache" when there really wasn't one, just so Mom would mix up the medicine.

She combined a half-glass of water, a half-glass of cider vinegar and enough sugar to sweeten. Last she added ¾ teaspoon of soda and stirred it to make it fizz.

We called this "vinegar whiz"— and it was a sure cure for the bellyache.

—**Gertrude Shoaf**

I will give you an old grandpa's remedy. I am 85 years old, so you can see what an old cold remedy can do:

Cut sassafras roots into small pieces, the more the better. Put them in a container of water and boil until the water changes color—then drink.

—**H.J. Benny**

I was born in 1906, and as I grew up there were many odd remedies on the home front. Some of them worked. Here are a few:

For colds and cough, Mom put a few drops of camphor on a sugar lump. I took it with no argument as I loved sweets in any form.

For a sore throat she rubbed my chest and

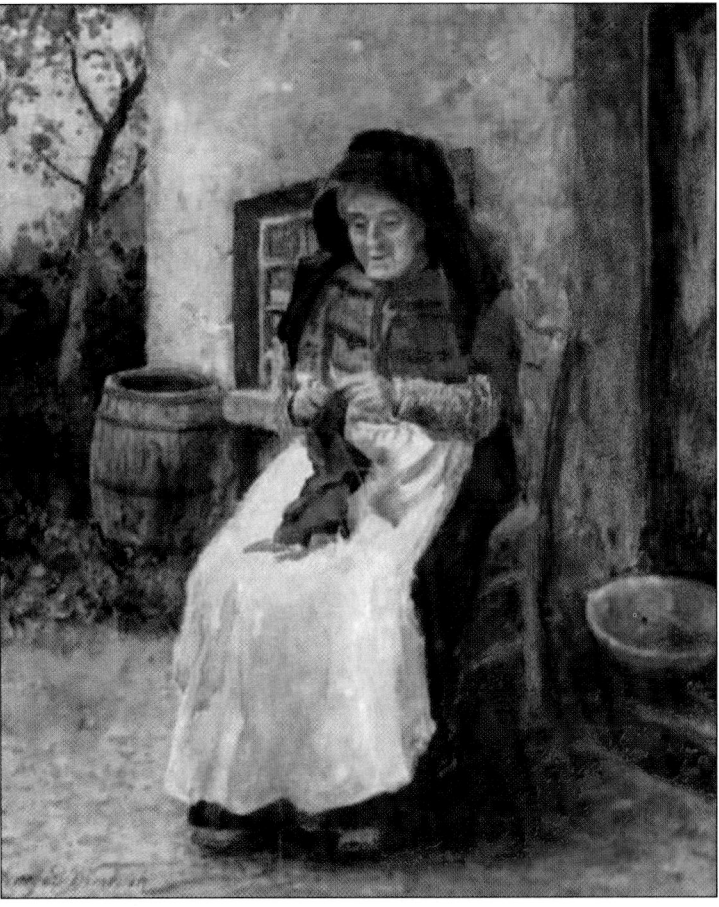

throat with goose grease saved from Thanksgiving and Christmas. Then she covered a red flannel cloth with the grease and turpentine and put that on my chest. I stayed in bed and played with her jewelry box.

For a cold she cooked honey, lemon juice and flaxseed together. I loved that mixture. She also gave me horehound drops which I gobbled as though they were candy. My colds never lasted long or caused any special trouble.

When I had one mild appendix attack she wrapped ice in a cloth and applied it to the area and it was soon forgotten. It remained for me to have a ruptured appendix just a few months ago, at age 80!

When I was hoarse I was given licorice. So I didn't mind being hoarse.

—**Marie Lundgren**

Cure-Alls for Kids

By Annabelle Scott Whobrey

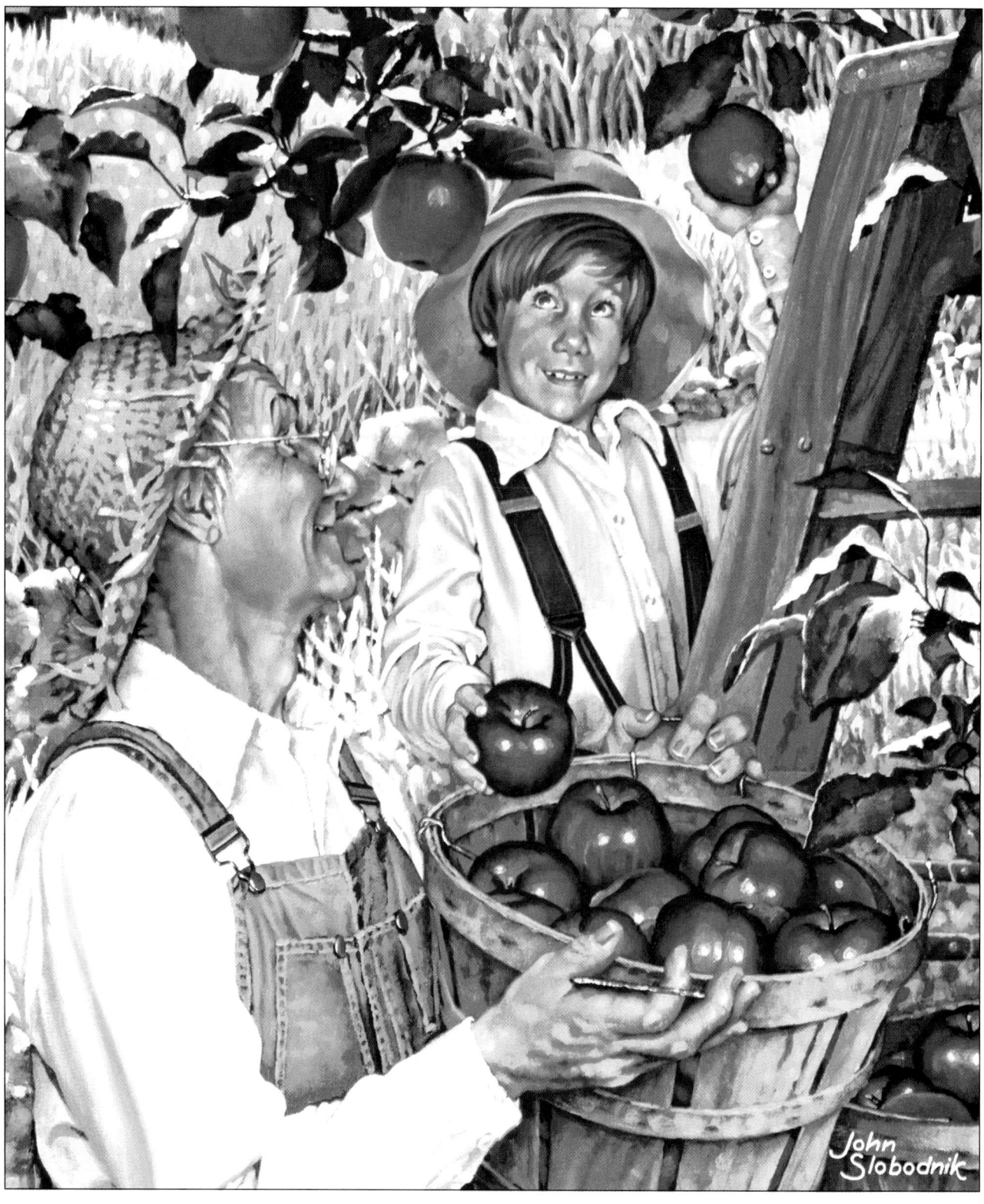

I wonder how in the wide world I ever lived to get grown? I was never rushed off to a doctor or given prescription medicine. Mama had a home remedy for anything that ailed me.

As soon as signs of fall began to appear, a round of turpentine treatment was a must! Many in Mama's family had died of typhoid fever and she wasn't about to risk her darling daughter getting the dread disease. Thus my yearly purging with her preventative.

No germ could have survived in the wake of that terrible-tasting turpentine. Goodness, I was belching it long after I donned long underwear! But Mama made my doses as pleasant as possible by putting the few drops of turpentine on a spoonful of sugar.

Mama also applied turpentine externally. If I stepped on a stub or broken glass, or jumped off a haystack and got a stone bruise, out came the turpentine! First the wound was soaked in a pan of coal oil, then it was bandaged in turpentine and sugar.

There were no neat Band-Aids, or even adhesive tape. Mama saved worn-out sheets and pillow cases, and when the need arose, "Florence Nightingale" was prepared! She used the oven of her wood-burning cookstove to sterilize the bandages, and wrapped my foot until it looked like a mummy's!

But don't think that was the end of her nursing—she kept a close watch for red streaks running from the wound. If any appeared, she filled the wash pan with very warm water and added half a cup of epsom salts, and I sat for hours, soaking out the infection.

Epsom salts had other redeeming qualities besides. When ponds and rivers got low during the summer drought, we all received doses of salts. Mama thought that mosquitoes injected malaria germs and prescribed these terrible-tasting salts. If one was unwilling to swallow the dose, then it was poured down his nose! This was crude, but it beat dying—or so Mama thought.

Today there are tests which can determine if a child has parasites. But Mama could tell when I was wormy by noting a white ring around my mouth. Then, off the shelf came the vermifuge. The results were gratifying—or so Mama said after closely observing her child.

I was a willing patient when it came to taking syrup of pepsin. I loved the stuff! In fact, I once downed a whole bottle. Mama up and called the family doctor, but he didn't get a bit excited; he said it wouldn't hurt me. He did give a bit of advice: "Don't keep any doors locked, so she can make a fast exit!"

My reaction to my overdose was similar to that to eating too many green apples. Our farm had apple trees, and as soon as they shed their blooms I began to hunt green apples to eat. Green apples sprinkled with salt and eaten high in a tree were quite the delicacy! But when I overindulged, Mama had the cure. She dropped some Raleigh's Red Liniment into a glass of warm water and sweetened it, and as I drank it I felt my tummy relax.

I was a willing patient when it came to taking syrup of pepsin. I loved it!

Every summer there seemed to be a "mad dog" scare. A strange-acting dog would wander through the community and everyone watched out for it for fear that it would bite their livestock, dogs or kids. We took precautions, because even Mama didn't have a remedy for hydrophobia. She knew where a cure was—in West Plains, but that was too far away. The "cure" was the breast bone of a white deer; when placed on the bite, it supposedly drew out the poison. Thanks to my guardian angel I never needed this "cure," and I'm sure it wouldn't have worked anyway. But I know Mama would have made every effort to try it!

Mama knew a sure-fire cure for a baby with colic. A tablespoon of warm coffee gave relief in no time. I acquired the coffee habit early in life, thanks to this remedy.

Old-timers had cure-alls for most any ailment. Now these have given way to modern medicine. Shots and pills have replaced Mama's home remedies. Even the "peach tree tea" she gave me for my bad temper has given way to books and talks on misbehavior. I can tell you one thing: her applications of "peach tree tea" on my backside were never forgotten! So, 70 years have updated the realm of the medical world— and Mama's methods of discipline! ◆

A Case of Mumps

By Dorothy Taylor

At the turn of the century in rural America, physicians were few and far between, and their services were sought mainly in times of crisis. Childhood diseases seldom required more than the attention of one's mother who, steeping in medical folklore, functioned as doctor and nurse with admirable success.

Because I was so miserably sick, I remember the mumps. A few days after Christmas I showed signs of an upset stomach with headache and fever. At first my symptoms seemed a casual holiday hangover attributed to excitement and overeating, but when large swellings appeared on both sides of my face, my mother said, "Why, you must have the mumps!"

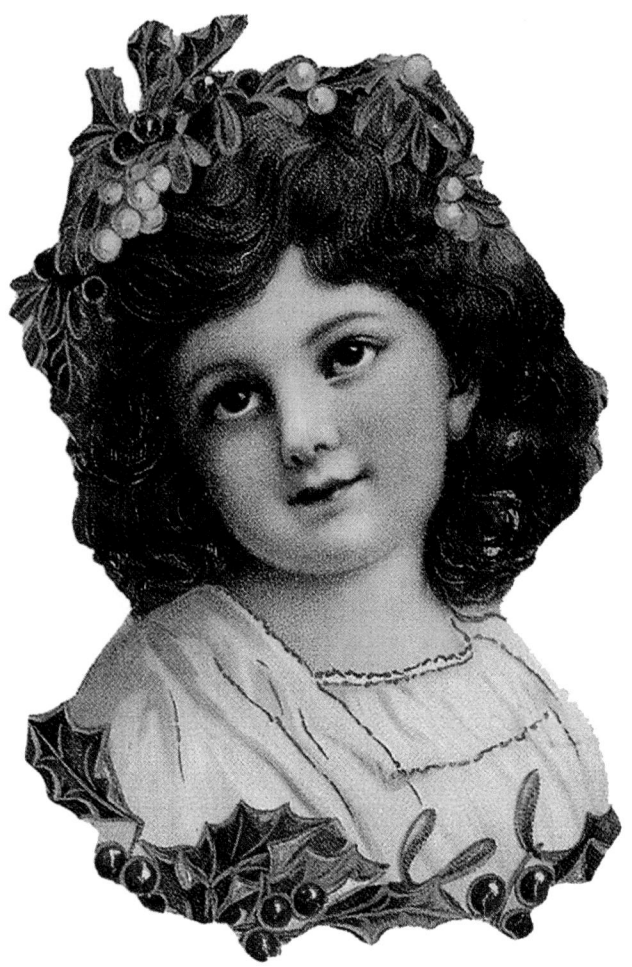

Immediate treatment consisted of applications of hot pancakes to the afflicted areas. My mother made delicious pancakes, and at any other time I would have teased for a stack smothered in butter and honey. But now I could not bear to look at food. The swelling persisted. The pancake treatment was a failure.

My mother, however, had other nostrums in her armamentarium. She boiled a pot of potatoes. I can see her still as she pounded them with a large wooden masher. She added huge lumps of butter and whipped the mixture to a creamy consistency. From her rag bag, she fetched a piece of soft flannel. She spread the mashed potatoes along its length, and after folding the cloth she applied this poultice to my face and throat with a secure knot on the top of my head.

The mashed potatoes appeared to do the trick. Each morning for several days my mother made fresh mashed potatoes. I wore the poultices without protest because the treatment seemed to help and I began to feel better.

My father, a railroader, was paid once a month. On payday my mother had to go to town to settle accounts and order supplies for the next few weeks. She decided I had recovered enough to be left alone. Before setting out, she applied my potato pack. I waved goodbye from the window.

During my illness I had eaten very little. Now I began to have visions of my mother's return from her shopping trip laden with goodies. I began to feel hungry.

The morning dragged along. My mother was late. I thought she would certainly bring me some honey jumble cookies, and there would be other things, too. Perhaps she would bring me a little bag of my favorite candies.

My goodness, how hungry I was! Finally, in desperation, I opened the poultice and ate the potatoes.

When my mother came home, she smiled and said I was cured. ◆

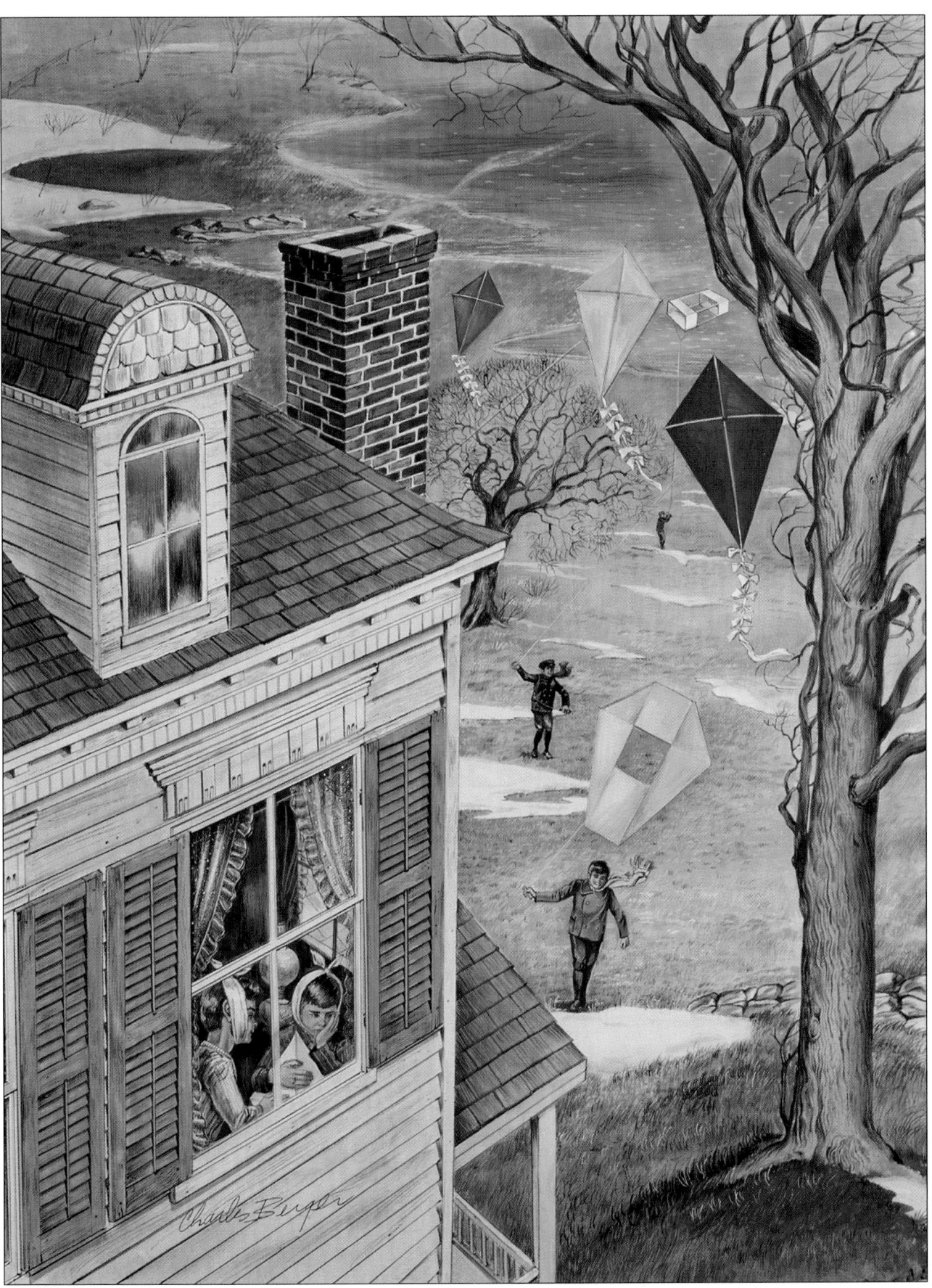

Papa's Remedies

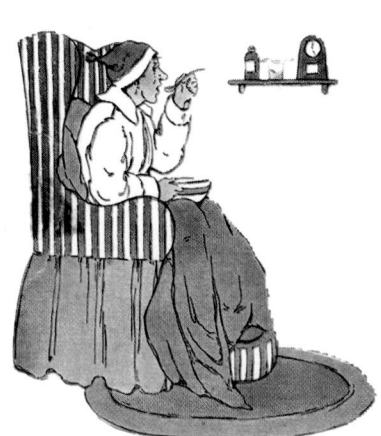

By Edna Barnes

My father was a man of unquestioned authority who taught with swift discipline. But when one of his family was ill, his heart quickly filled with compassion. However, during an epidemic in our small town in Jefferson County, Nebr., during the winter of 1915–1916, his unyielding attitude backfired.

Papa had a remedy for everything—that is, by his own diagnosis. Like his Pennsylvania Dutch ancestors, he depended largely on nature's cures for each ailment. It was surprising how often these remedies worked; we seldom needed a doctor's services.

Papa had a system for treating sore throats. We children went first to Mama, who measured out a teaspoon of sugar. Then Papa would add a drop or two of coal oil. The mixture wasn't hard to swallow, but the taste lingered for a long time.

For a more severe sore throat, an onion poultice was applied. Onions were baked in their skins on the hearth of the wood-burning stove. Then they were wrapped in a woolen sock and wrapped around the neck.

When I was 8, I had a throat so sore that it didn't respond to any of Papa's remedies. An epidemic of diphtheria threatened our area, causing my parents a great deal of concern. Remembering the test his mother had used, Papa set about to diagnose my case. He inserted the handle of a silver spoon down my throat; it was most unpleasant. If the spoon turned green, he knew there would be cause for alarm. That test satisfied him that mine was simply a stubborn sore throat which needed additional home treatment.

The next step was to give me Carter's Little Liver Pills. Try as I might, I couldn't make myself swallow that little red pill. Papa tried to make me forget it with his little tricks. Still, it showed up on the end of my tongue.

Finally Papa brought a pitcher of cream. Pouring a teaspoonful, he said, "Here, take this and the pill will slide down."

I swallowed one spoonful after another, but the pill stayed put. Papa coaxed and cajoled until finally he became exasperated. Turning to Mama, he sighed and said, "Just like my mother; she couldn't swaller a pill to save her life."

That did it! I knew Grandma had died. Was it because she couldn't

Papa had a system for treating sore throats. The mixture wasn't hard to swallow, but the taste lingered for a long time.

swallow a pill? That little pill disappeared so quickly that it frightened me. Next morning, Papa said I was "outta the woods" and could return to school soon.

One quiet night while we were all sleeping, my 12-year-old sister, Mabel, startled us by screaming. She jumped out of the blanket up to the bedstead as if trying to climb the wall! Her feet dancing and shaking, she jabbered in quick breaths, uttering unintelligible sounds. Her actions scared me so that I sat up in bed and yelled, "Mabel's having a fit!"

Our parents were in our room in a flash! Mama sat on the bed, took Mabel on her lap and spoke softly to quiet her. Papa diagnosed it in one word: "Worms!" He went to the kitchen and returned with a spoonful of sugar. "To feed 'em," he explained. Mama preferred to think it had been a bad dream, but Papa's pride was preserved and we all settled down.

Of all Papa's remedies, his "private medicine" concerned Mama most. One evening Papa came home late, running the horses in high gear and lifting his voice to the sky, singing *In the Sweet Bye and Bye.*

It was a still night, and we could hear him from the time he left town almost a mile away. While we waited supper, we listened to his song blend with the rattle of the wagon and the jangle of the harness. The two older boys lit lanterns and waited for him.

Louder and louder his voice became, reaching a crescendo as the horses turned down the driveway. Mother went out to help him down from the wagon and into the house. He stopped to lean against the long dining table, staring with red, glassy eyes at the little ones who scampered for cover. His ability to frighten them caused a burst of laughter.

Mama tucked him into bed. Then one of the younger ones asked, "What's the matter with Papa?"

"Hush!" she said with a wave of her hand. "Papa's full. He took too much medicine. Be quiet and let him sleep."

In addition to the diphtheria, some small-pox cases began to appear. Health officials were concerned that another epidemic might be forth-coming. Teachers sent forms home with the students to get their parents' signatures so they could receive vac-cinations as protec-tion against the disease.

"No!" Papa was emphatic. "It's just horse serum. What good'll that do ya?"

"But, but …" I tried to interrupt. Papa put his big hand on my mouth.

"I'm agin it, I said! I heard folks got vaccinated and gotta worse kinda case. Tell yer teacher I do not b'lieve in it! You won't git it if yer not around it. Just keep wearin' that asafetida on yer neck—it'll ward off anything."

"Even my friends," I muttered under my breath.

I was embarrassed to hand in the unsigned form. I put the paper on Miss Major's desk with-out looking up. Starting to my seat, I turned to see Miss Major give me a second glance and I heard her sigh as she picked up the paper. I sensed that she'd gotten a whiff of the fetid resin.

She quickly turned her attention to the desk.

A few days later Papa surprised us by coming home early. He was accompanied by a deputy sheriff who carried a large red-and-black sign. We read the bold letters: "SMALLPOX." It frightened us to see the deputy tack the sign onto our house. We had seen such a sign on our neighbor's house and we walked in the street when we went by to avoid getting too close to the house. Now that quarantine sign was on our home!

Papa had a remedy for everything— that is, by his own diagnosis. He depended largely on nature's cures.

The deputy turned and gave us instructions. "Don't leave this yard nor have any company for three weeks. Understand?"

We nodded.

This unscheduled vacation put us in a hilarious mood. We whooped and hollered in the yard, jumping around like Indians in a war dance. Our noise brought a neighbor to the back fence. "What are you celebrating?" she inquired. "Why aren't you in school?"

Suddenly we struck a dead silence; then we started snickering. Finally little Ted piped up. "Papa's got smallpox!"

She backed away from the fence as if she had been struck. Without a word or even a look back at us, she ran into her house. We children doubled up with laughter.

Papa had known little sickness in his life, so he groaned and complained. Ted, not yet 3, heard Papa moan that he was dying. Cautiously he opened the bedroom door and peeped in. Then he ran in! Holding out his fetid wad on a string, he cried, "Here, Pap, you take my 'sfety."

"No, Baby, you keep it. I already got 'em. Yer Papa's awful sick."

Putting his little arms around Papa's neck, Ted cried as if his heart were broken. Suddenly he released his grip and turned toward the door, sobbing, "Mama can git you some hoss serp." He bolted toward the kitchen where he buried

his head in her long skirt. She stroked his curly red hair while she reassured him with a piece of warm bread.

Perhaps someone should have reassured the young man who brought the first delivery. He drove a one-horse vehicle. Seeing the sign on the house, he didn't drop the tether to hold the horse. Instead he tossed the packages by the gate, gave a furtive glance at the house, and leaped back onto the moving wagon like a pony express rider.

By the time Papa recovered others were getting the disease. But our sleeping habits hadn't changed. As usual, I slept with Mabel, who was very ill. Yet I was spared. Mother also stayed well, and she and I worked together to care for the five others in bed.

On the day Papa no longer needed to be quarantined he was met on the back porch by an official from the health department who sprayed him and the contents of his valise. Now he was quarantined *out*. He could bring our supplies and leave them at the gate, but he was not allowed to enter. We watched from the window for his arrival, then stepped out onto the cold porch to throw kisses. After he left we raced to pick up the packages.

Ted, though last to get the disease, became critically ill. Mama was so concerned that she called Papa, who notified the doctor. Shortly after that the doctor arrived at the house and treated our youngest brother, who soon recovered.

When the quarantine was finally lifted and the sign removed, the house had to be vacated all day for fumigation. We were invited to our neighbor's who had recovered from the disease earlier.

When we went home at dusk, the peppery odor of the gas from the burned formaldehyde candles still reeked in the cold air from open windows and doors.

Papa came. Leaving his horses standing in the yard, he leaped over the wagon wheel and ran into the house. Mama met him at the door and they shared a long embrace.

The next time a communicable disease threatened, Papa was the first to recommend vaccinations. ◆

My Father, The Dentist

By Doris Patterson

Well, actually, my father was a truck driver, but he did pull most of his nine children's loose teeth.

I remember how excited I'd be when I discovered a loose tooth. I would run to meet my father when he got home after a hard day at work. But instead of greeting him with "Hi, Daddy!" I'd ask, "Guess what?" and open my mouth much wider than was necessary. Then I'd wiggle the loose tooth with my finger—and soon Dad would have another "operation" to perform.

My dad must have grown weary of hearing the same question night after night and having to look in my mouth; sometimes he would sneak in the back door. The day of days would eventually arrive, though. The tooth was ready, I was ready, and by that time, Daddy was ready to pull any tooth that moved.

My father's "dental office" was his and my mother's bedroom. My brothers and sisters would stand by the door to give me all the support I needed, or to run for some tissue in case I needed that. I would stand in the middle of the room by the bed, under the chandelier.

"Open wide," my dentist father would say. "Hold your head way back. Don't move."

Before I knew what had happened, the tooth would be out and the only thing I felt was bits of coal from my father's hands. "Go wash your mouth out with warm salt water," he would say

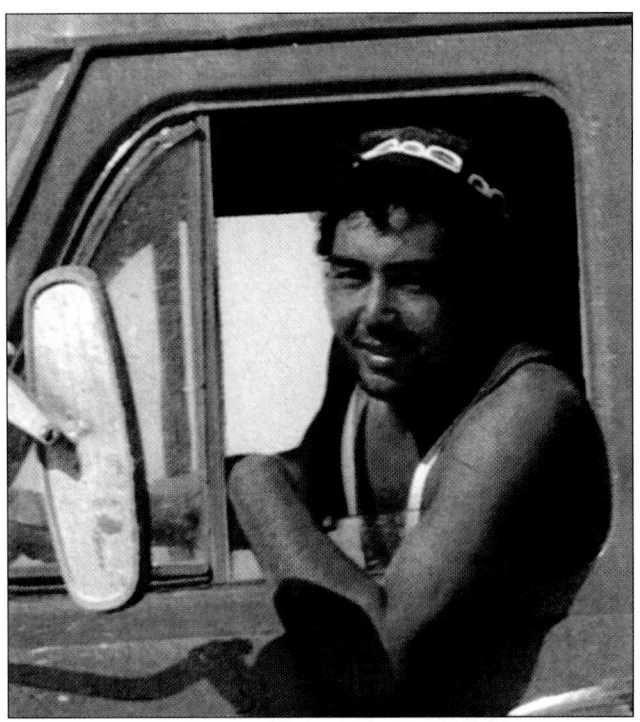

My father was actually a truck driver, but he did pull most of his nine children's teeth.

with orthodontic authority. Obediently, I would go to the bathroom, clutching the tooth in my hot little hand, to follow the instructions of my father, the dentist. ◆

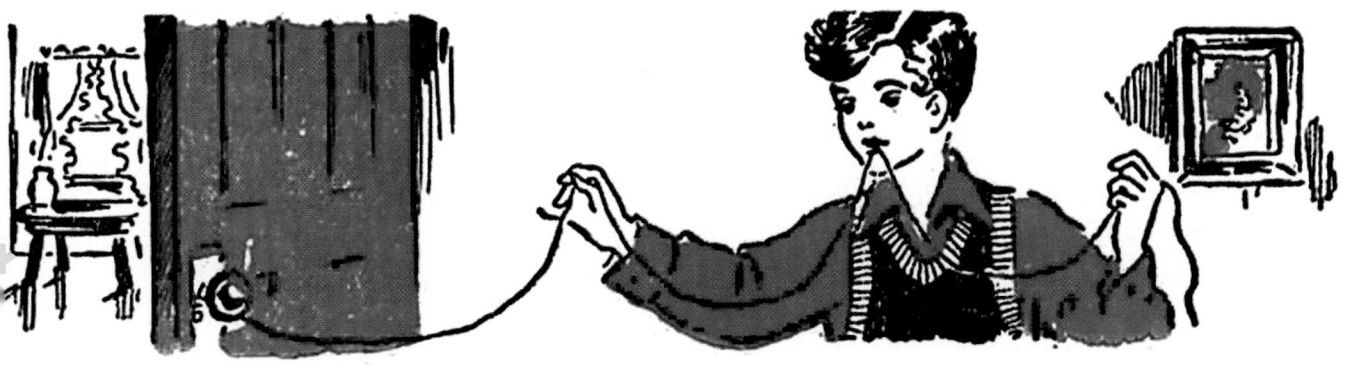

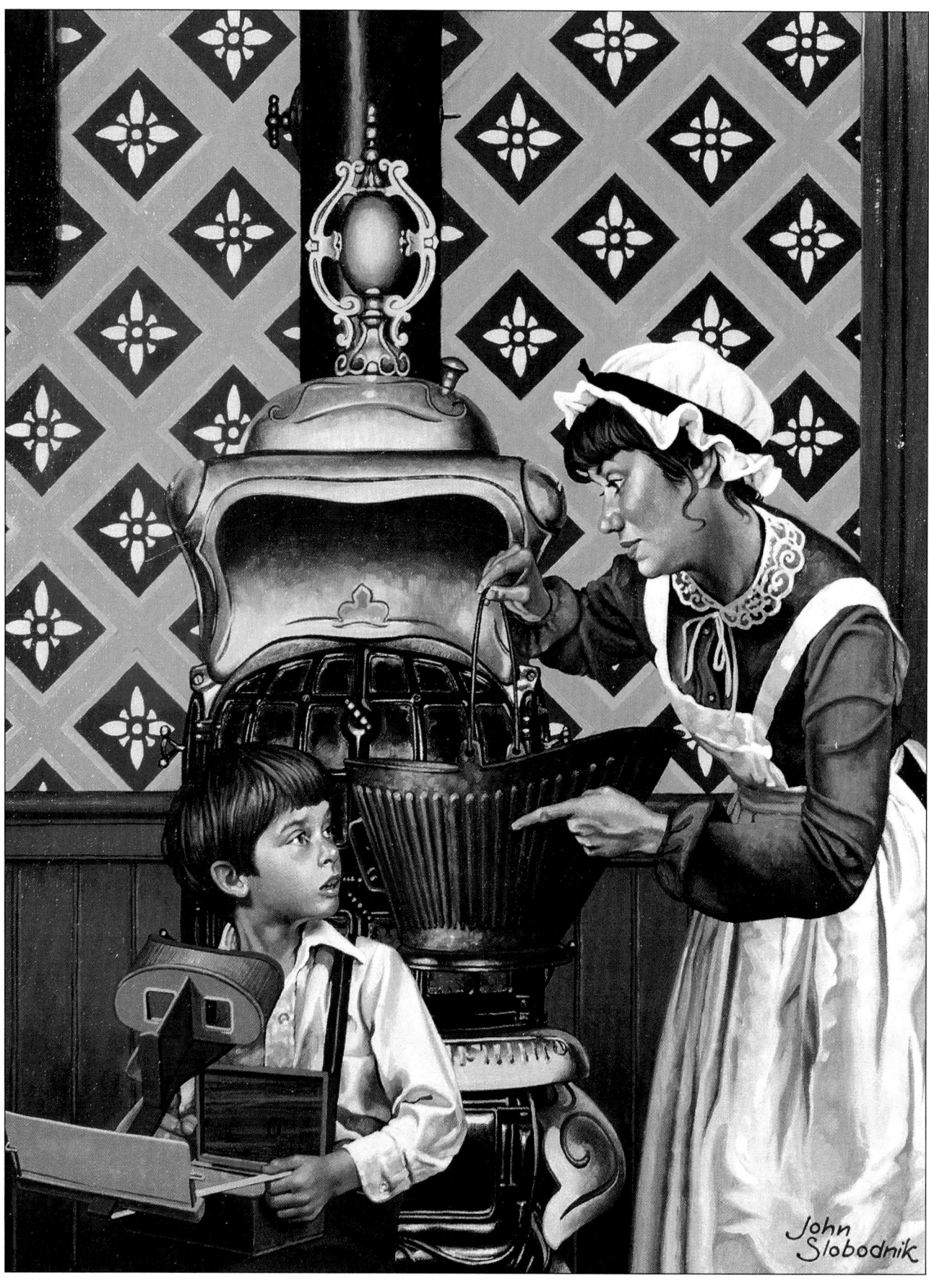

Home Remedies From 1896

Spice poultices: 1 tablespoonful of ground spice, 1 of black pepper, 1 of cloves and 1 of ginger mixed together in a bowl; put in a flannel bag and quilt across twice each way to keep it in place; sew up the end, wet with alcohol, heat and apply; save the bag and use when needed.

Wood ashes: Pour 1 pint of boiling water over 2 heaping tablespoonfuls of clean hard wood ashes; let it settle and cool, pour off the top and strain and put in a bottle. Instead of dosing with drugs when you have acidity of the stomach, take a spoonful of this weak lye.

A physician was sent for in great haste to attend a child who was subject to worm fits; he had driven several miles and found the child very sick with all the symptoms of worms. He ordered boiling water, prepared some wood ashes and poured the water over it; as soon as it cooled he gave the child 2 or 3 teaspoonfuls. The child was soon relieved.

Preventing a sty: Put 2 teaspoonsful of black tea in a small cheesecloth bag, put in a tin cup and pour enough boiling water over it to moisten it well; let it stand a few minutes. At night lay it over the eye where the sty is coming and let it remain there all night. If no better, apply the second night and wet the sty with some of the tea; it generally cures if taken in time.

A hot-water cure: A businessman who had chronic dyspepsia and was given up as incurable resolved to try the simple remedy of taking a cupful of hot water before breakfast every morning for three or four weeks. He sipped it with a spoon, as it was too hot to drink; at the end of four weeks he was so much better that he could eat any food that others could, had gained in weight and was cured of dyspepsia.

To make people plump: To a teacupful of hot water add 1 spoonful of sweet cream and drink half an hour before breakfast. It aids digestion and makes one plump.

Cough remedy: Cook 3 tablespoonsful of flaxseed, unground, in 1 quart of water. Strain; add some loaf sugar and a half a teacupful of honey and the juice of 3 or 4 lemons. Cook together and bottle for use. At night take half a cupful hot.

Old remedies for everything from coughs to constipation

For a cold: Put ¼ teaspoonful of cayenne pepper in a teacup. Pour over it a cupful of hot water. Sweeten with loaf sugar or honey. Strain and drink.

Brief Hints

For constipation, drink a glass of hot water with a spoonful of wheat bran stirred in it every morning.

For a puncture wound from a nail in the foot, apply a piece of salt pork and bind it on the foot, and keep the foot at rest on a chair or a stool for several days, if need be, to avoid inflammation and possible lock-jaw.

Burns: The white of an egg applied to a burn relieves the pain.

To prevent the skin from being discolored after a bruise, apply salt butter quickly. Very hot bathing of the part is also efficacious.

Insect bites: Borax is excellent for the bites of insects, as it neutralizes their acid properties.

Bee stings: Mud or clay is good to relieve a bee sting. Make it stiff and apply.

Earache is very painful. A dust of ground black pepper put in a dry piece of cotton wool and covered with the cotton, inserted in the ear, gives relief.

For erysipelas, a poultice made of pounded cranberries and applied is an excellent and safe remedy. ◆

Preventative Medicine

By June Masters Bacher

An ounce of prevention is worth a pound of cure." Gram'ma said that so often that the family grew to believe she was the first to come up with the truism. Maybe she was....

The eldest son was in medical school and the two of them kept a steady flow of written conversation going. Just how much she learned from him—or he from her!—is difficult to ascertain. Gram'ma always said that they learned from each other, "combining book learning and horse sense." Be that as it may, the chapter she recorded in her daily household diary-type ledger entitled "Health Suggestions" was one of her most eloquent.

"A great many cannot see why it is that they do not take a cold when exposed to cold winds and rain," she wrote on Jan. 12, 1887. She went on to explain the "facts."

"The fact is, and ought to be more generally understood, that nearly every cold is contracted indoors, and is not directly due to the cold outside but to the heat inside. A man will go to bed at night feeling as well as usual and get up in the morning with a royal cold. He goes peeking around in search of cracks and keyholes and tiny drafts. Weather strips are procured, and the house made as tight as a fruit can. In a few days more, the whole family has colds—worse ones!

"Let a man go home, tired, eat a big supper of starchy foods, occupy his mind intently too long, go to bed in a closed room in which there is no ventilation, and if he doesn't have a cold in the morning, there is something wrong with him.

"People swallow more colds down their throats than they inhale, no matter how chilly. Plain, light suppers are good to sleep on and more conducive to refreshing sleep than a glass of beer or dose of chloral. In the estimation of many, this is rank heresy, but in the light of science,

common sense, and experience, it is the gospel truth. Close foul air causes blood poisoning. It is estimated that a person corrupts one gallon of pure air every minute, or twenty-five barrels full in a single night, in breathing alone.

"In passing from warm crowded rooms to cold air, the mouth should be kept closed, and all the breathing done through the nostrils only, that the cold air may be warmed before it reaches the lungs....

"Beings need drink as much as food; and it is just as necessary as pure air; therefore, the water should be boiled. Rain water is the best.

"Water has other uses, too. For bruises, if applied at once, the use of hot water will generally prevent, nearly, if not entirely, the bruised flesh from turning black. For colic, sip a cupful of hot water. If that is insufficient, a flannel cloth folded in several thicknesses, large enough to fully cover the painful place, should be wrung out of hot water and laid over the seat of the pain. All in all, this is how to keep well: don't sleep in a draught; don't go to bed with cold feet; don't stand over hot-air registers; don't eat what you do not need, just save it; don't cool too quickly; don't sleep without ventilation; don't stuff a cold lest you should be next obliged to starve a fever; don't sit in a damp room without a fire; and don't try to get along without flannel underwear during the dead of winter.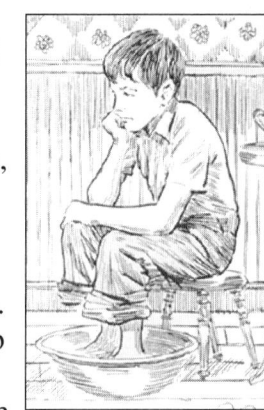

"If you take precautions and still you catch a cold from another there is still hope to be had in cures. For sudden hoarseness, beat the white of an egg, add the juice of one lemon, sweeten with honey and take a teaspoonful. Try baking a lemon twenty minutes in a moderate oven. When done, open at one end and sweeten with molasses. Be sure to soak the feet in hot mustard water each night."

The "lady doctor" of more than a century ago summarized: "All in all, it seems easier to prevent a cold than to cure one." Perhaps that was the wisest of all my grandmother's prescriptions! ◆

Mama Cleaned Us Out

By Ruth M. Outwater

Mama considered food to be the panacea for all ills of the human spirit. When Buddy or I was bored, unhappy, quarrelsome or just not feeling up to snuff, she'd say, "You're probably hungry. You will feel better after you have something to eat." And sure enough, a slice of bread with butter and sugar, or a glass of milk with a couple of Dutch boy cookies, would bring marked improvement. Dutch boy cookies were round, flat sugar cookies with a hole in the middle and scallops around the edge. The only acceptable way to eat them, of course, was to stick your finger through the hole and nibble around the edge until there was nothing left but a ring on your finger.

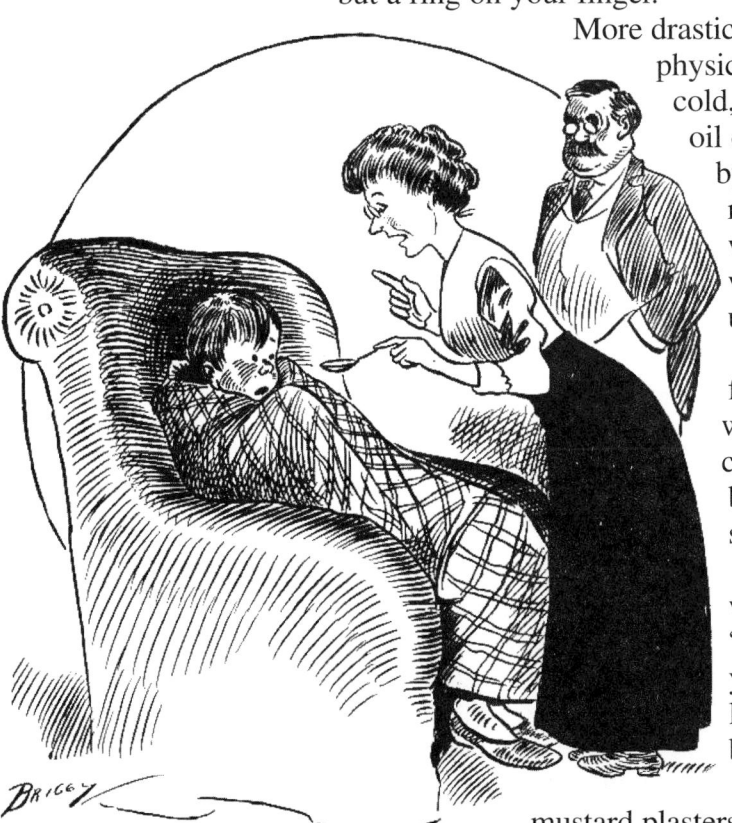

More drastic measures were required in the case of physical ailments. Every time one of us had a cold, the whole house reeked of camphorated oil or mustard plasters or both. Mama swore by these time-tested remedies, but the only reason Buddy and I didn't swear *at* them was because we didn't know any swear words. We wouldn't have been allowed to use them anyway.

We had other ways of making our feelings known. Seeing Mama coming with a saucer of warm oil and a flannel cloth, the invalid would pull the bedclothes over his or her head and scream hoarsely, "Take it away! It stinks!"

"Now that isn't a nice word," Mama would admonish, pulling back the covers. "Besides, this doesn't smell bad at all. Do you know what Grandma did when I was a little girl? She made me wear an asafetida bag around my neck. *That* really smelled!"

We objected just as strongly to the mustard plasters. Even before the cold, clammy thing had begun to warm up, we'd be yelling in agony. "Take it off! Quick! It's burning!"

Poor Mama, just to make sure, would lift one corner of the plaster and say, "Why, your skin isn't even pink yet! Do you know what Grandma did when I was a little girl and had tonsillitis? (These questions of Mama's were purely rhetorical; she expected no answer from us but always provided her own.) She tied strips of raw bacon fat around my neck. That was a *lot* worse than mustard plasters!"

A man from the health department was always tacking a quarantine sign on our front door. We kept getting the same diseases over and over.

The only thing that made life bearable when we had colds was the flaxseed tea Mama made with honey and lemon juice which she gave us for our coughs. This was perfectly delicious— much better than candy—and it was surprising how long our coughs hung on sometimes.

A man from the health department was always tacking a quarantine sign on our front door. It wasn't that we went in for a variety of diseases; we kept getting the same ones over and over. We had red measles, German measles, three-day measles and chicken pox twice. I was the one who brought these germs into the house, and it wasn't until I had been pro- nounced cured and fit to be turned loose in society once more that Buddy would "break out"—and back would come the man from the health department.

Mama worried about the effect measles might have on our eyes. When that disease was present, she protected us from the light by keeping the green roller shades pulled down and pinning newspaper to the lace curtains. In the evenings the dangling electric bulbs wore little newspaper bags. During the long, itchy nights of chicken pox, Mama was always there when we called her, her hand cool on our burning foreheads, rubbing zinc ointment on our spots.

As I was considered a sickly child, I was

always being dosed with something or other. Mama would start out hopefully by trying to make a game of it. "Open your mouth and close your eyes, I'll give you something to make you wise," she'd say mysteriously, then pop a spoonful of some vile-tasting brew into my wide-open mouth.

But even a dullard like me could not be fooled indefinitely by this approach. Mama soon learned to give liquid medication in the kitchen whenever possible, as it was easier to wipe up spots from the linoleum than to wash the sheets and blankets. These occasions would find me hopping from one foot to the other and Mama standing in front of me with a spoonful of medicine and a glass of water. "I can't take it," I'd cry, making retching sounds. "It's nasty!"

"You haven't tasted it yet," she would say, a note of exasperation in her voice. "Do you know what Grandma made me take when I was a little girl? Sulphur and molasses! I would never give you anything that tasted *that* bad!"

After awhile I'd manage to squeeze my eyes shut, hold my nose and open my mouth as wide as it would go. But just as Mama would get the spoon to my lips, I'd jerk back convulsively, sending the spoon and its contents flying across the room.

When it came to patience, Mama could have taught Job a thing or two.

Our neighbor Mrs. Fraser, being the wife of a doctor, felt herself qualified to make what she called "iron pills." She gave a supply to Mama, assuring her that they were just the thing for what ailed me. These greenish-black pills, about the size of a large marble, were of a gelatin consistency, soft to the touch, and they stank to high heaven. Mrs. Fraser hadn't yet mastered the art of sugar-coating her wares, and I found it absolutely impossible to swallow one without it sticking halfway down my throat. I made such a "fuss and holler"—much worse than usual— that one day Mama said, in desperation, "Here! I'll take one and show you how easy it is!" After that I never had to take another iron pill.

Buddy did not have all this trouble swallowing medicine. The thing that would send him running through the house looking for

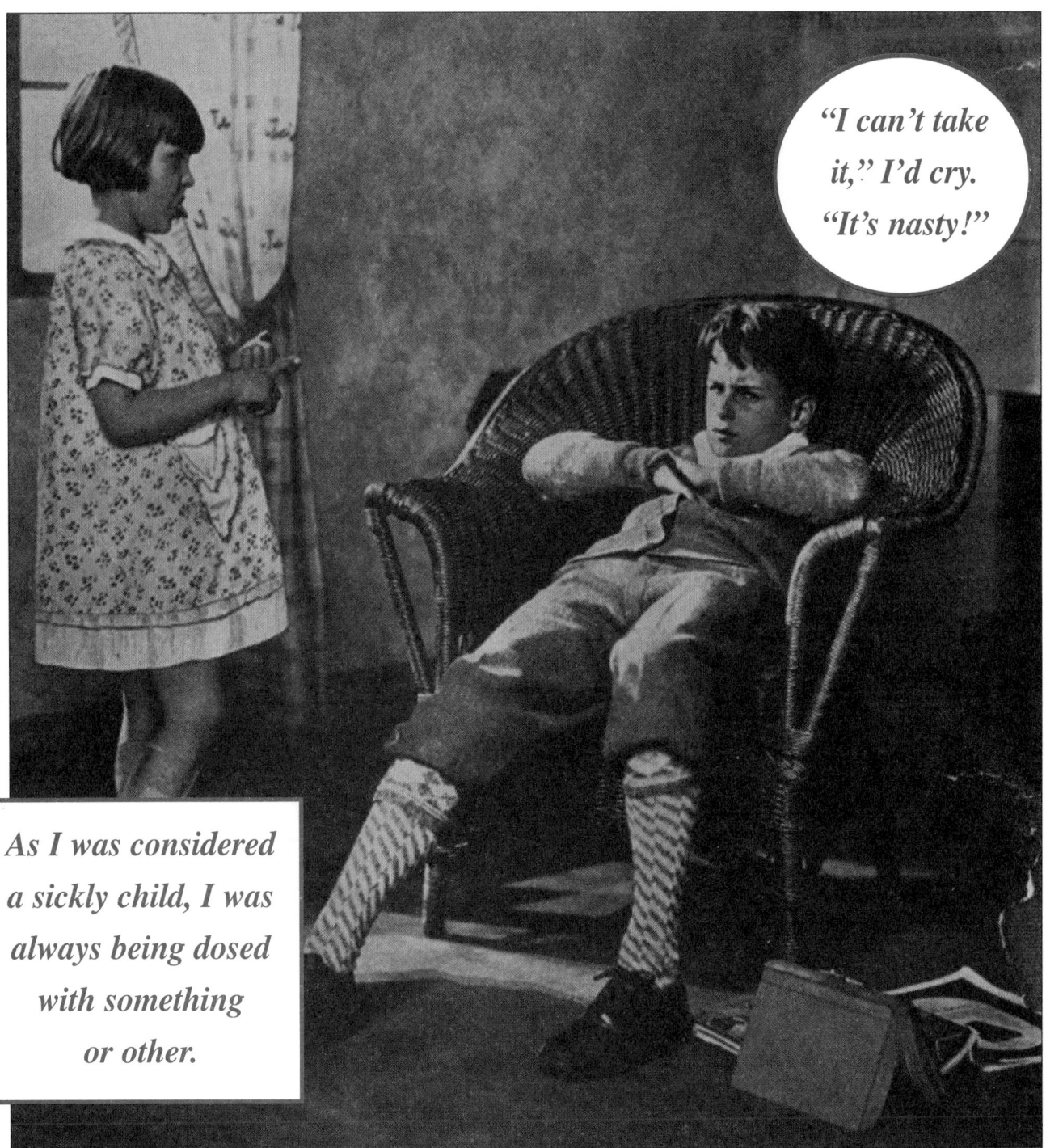

"I can't take it," I'd cry. "It's nasty!"

As I was considered a sickly child, I was always being dosed with something or other.

a hiding place was what he and Mama referred to as "the enemy." Even when we were feeling fine, Mama might look at us thoughtfully and decide we needed "a good cleaning out."

The most potent agency ever devised for this purpose was Calomel. The small white tablets looked innocent enough, but they contained the force of atomic energy. We were given two tablets at three- or four-hour intervals during the day, the last dose topped off with a brimming glass of citrate of magnesia. By then we were too sick to hold our heads up. The cleaning out that followed shortly thereafter was so complete and utterly overwhelming that, by comparison, camphorated oil and mustard plasters were fun. ◆

Mother Had The Remedy

By Davene Dority

When we were sick, Mother had a cure for everything. During the winter, when one of us woke with a cough or a hoarse throat, she would jump out of bed, light the oil lamp and head for the "hogfoot oil."

When we killed hogs, the feet were boiled and the oil was poured into a bottle. Mother would pour some of the oil into a teaspoon, hold it over the lighted lamp and let it warm and melt enough for us to swallow. We didn't dare cough again, lest we had to undergo another dose of that dreadful stuff. And, oh yes, it was good for earaches, too.

For sore throats we were given a teaspoon of sugar with two or three drops of turpentine. When we were unfortunate enough to suffer with chills and fever, she went for the Groves Tasteless Chill Tonic. If *that* was tasteless, God forbid that I should ever have to take anything with taste! We took five doses the first day, then waited three days. If no more chills or fever occurred, we were pronounced well. However, if we did chill again on the third day, it was back to square one.

In 1937, while my dad's brother was living with us and going to school, he came down with pneumonia. The doctor came to our house and stayed day and night for several days.

During that time, my sister Katherine also developed pneumonia. For days we weren't sure whether they would make it or not.

We lived in a 10-room house, so members of Dad's and Mom's families were able to come and help out. Neighbors came in to clean up—and someone always had to be with the sick. All night, the adults worked in shifts. Pallets were spread all over the floors and we slept wherever we could find a space.

The patient couldn't be permitted to get cold, so pots of water were kept on the old wood-burning stove so there would be plenty of hot water to refill the hot water bottles (glass jars wrapped in towels) around the patients' bodies.

It was believed then that the ninth day of an illness was the turning point, when the patient would either get much better, or take a turn for

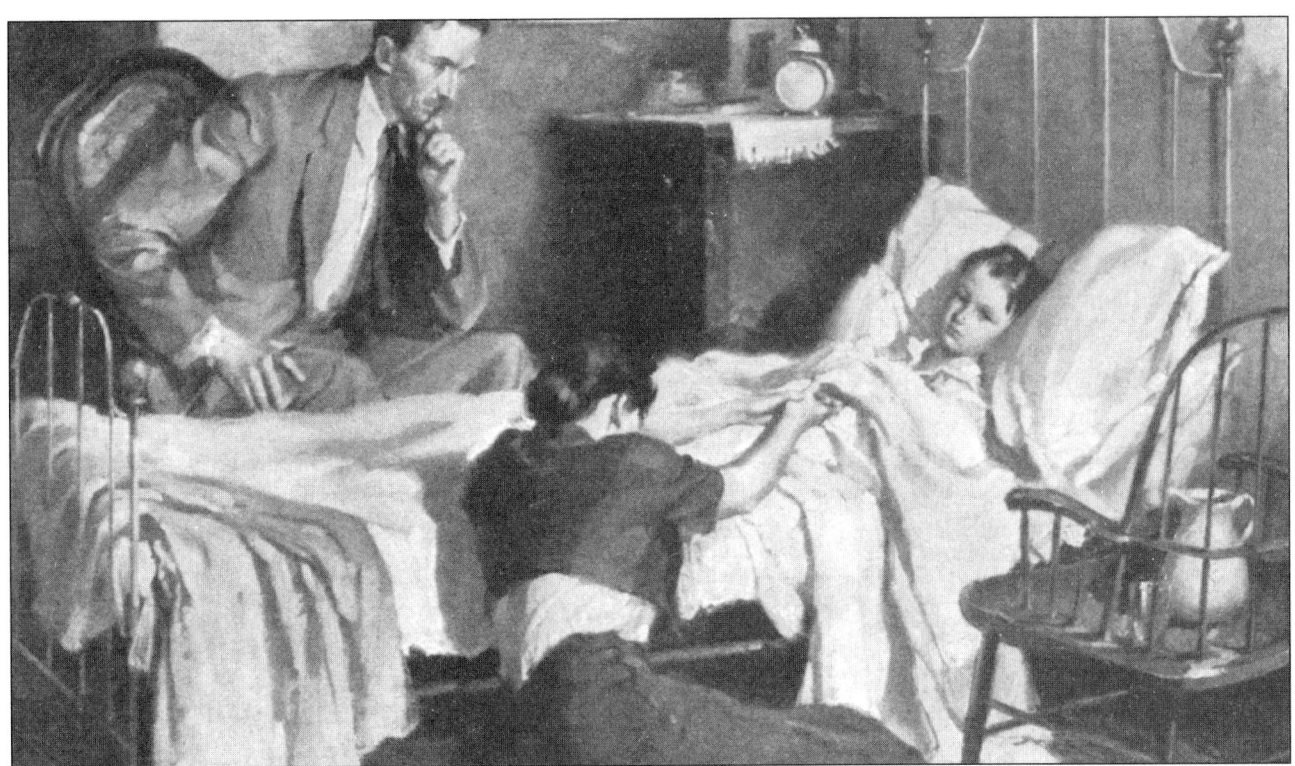

the worse and eventually die. My grandmother stayed in bed with Katherine all day to give her added body warmth. It was a long, somber day; everyone was unusually quiet and much prayer was offered to God.

Thankfully, they both made it and returned to good health. Everyone went home and our lives returned to normal. I was glad to get my bed back.

When the itch came to our school, our mother made sure there was enough hot water for the three of us to take a bath in Lysol water immediately after we came in from school. It worked—we never had the itch.

When we cut ourselves, Mother poured turpentine over the cut or, better still, made us soak the cut in kerosene.

I was a clumsy person, so it wasn't unusual for me to have a sprained arm or ankle. Mother made a poultice of clay and vinegar, put that all over the injury, wrapped it and left it wrapped for days. This kept the arm or ankle from swelling.

We three kids were healthy, but Mother had the idea that to keep us healthy, we had to take medicine every six months to flush malaria out of our systems. She gave us a medicine called Calomel. We took three pills a day for five days, then flushed medicine and malaria out with a castor oil laxative. Never has there ever been such an ordeal in the name of health!

Anyway, she gave Terrell and Katherine their castor oil first because they were no problem. I was a different story. She would pull a chair up beside my bed and tell me that if I didn't take the castor oil and flush out my body, my tongue would rot off. I tried, but as soon as I smelled the oil, I gagged. Then she pleaded and begged, but I just couldn't take it. Finally she got around to offering me money, and I would hold my nose and take the oil, simply declaring that I was going to die. That was the worst medicine ever made by God or man!

One day I made the mistake of telling her that my right side really hurt. She said, "Sis, if you will take it, I will mix you something to cure it."

She was so sincere that I said, "Fix it and I will take it." She did. It was a glass of buttermilk, orange juice and *castor oil*. I drank it, and believe it or not, the pain did go away— or maybe I was just too scared to admit that the pain was still there.

I am 69 years old now and even today, when I mention an ailment, Mother has a remedy. But I can't complain, because I am in great health. ◆

The Fragrance of Roses

By Evelyn Witter

Almost everyone loves the fragrance of roses. You can save that fragrance by saving the rose petals in a rose jar. Rose jars were popular before the days of air fresheners in aerosol cans.

To make a rose jar, find a good-looking jar with a loose-fitting lid. The jar can be pottery, porcelain or china.

Gather petals early in the morning about the time the dew is gone.

Spread the petals on absorbent paper in the shade. Allow them to dry for an hour or so; then, spread a half-inch layer of petals in a bowl.

Sprinkle the layer of petals lightly with table salt.

Day after day, add additional petals which have been handled in the same manner until, when they are pressed together firmly, they are the thickness of two quarters.

Each day, stir the petals in the bowl thoroughly.

Ten days after you've made the last addition, stir them thoroughly; then …

In a separate container, mix the following materials which can be obtained at the grocery and drugstore: ¼ ounce each of ground mace, cloves and allspice; ½ ounce ground cinnamon; 2 ounces powdered orris root; and 4 ounces dried lavender leaves.

Combine mixture with rose petals and place in the rose jar. Remember that the rose jar may be an attractive jar of your choosing, but it must have a lid to keep the aroma from escaping until you want it. When you want to enjoy the scent of roses in your room, just remove the lid and your room will soon have a sweet, old-fashioned fragrance that will delight you. ◆

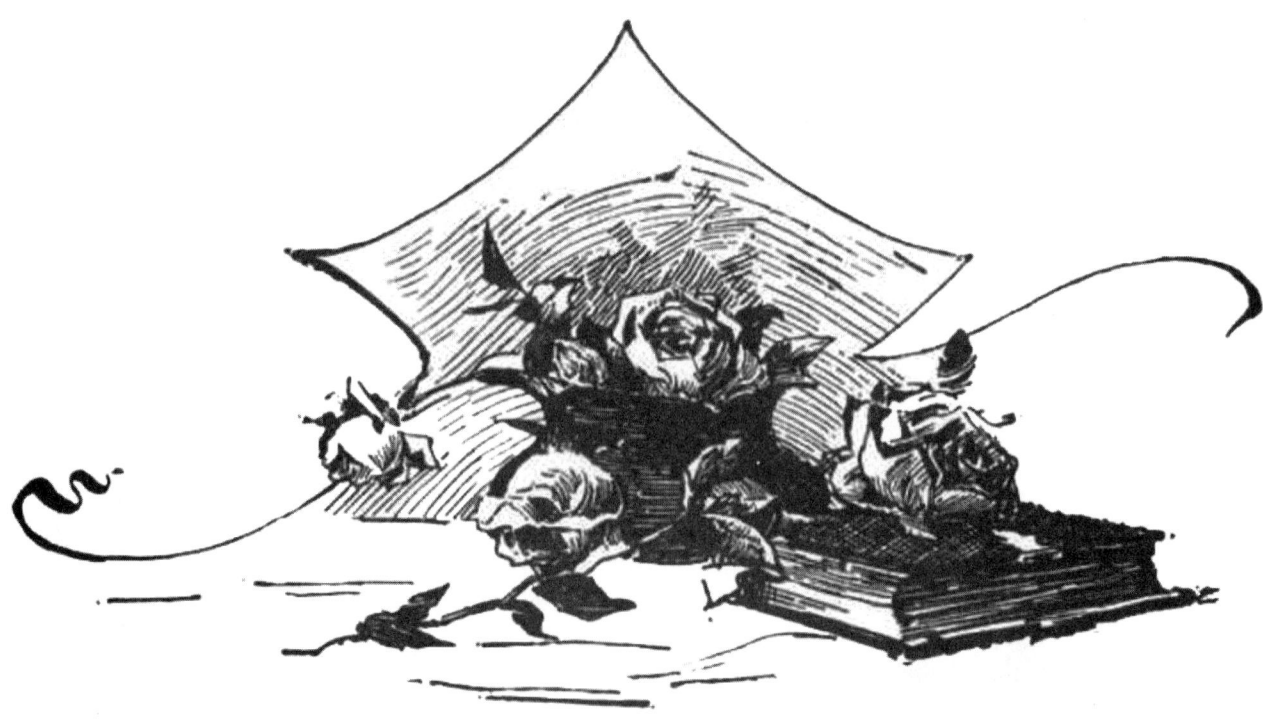

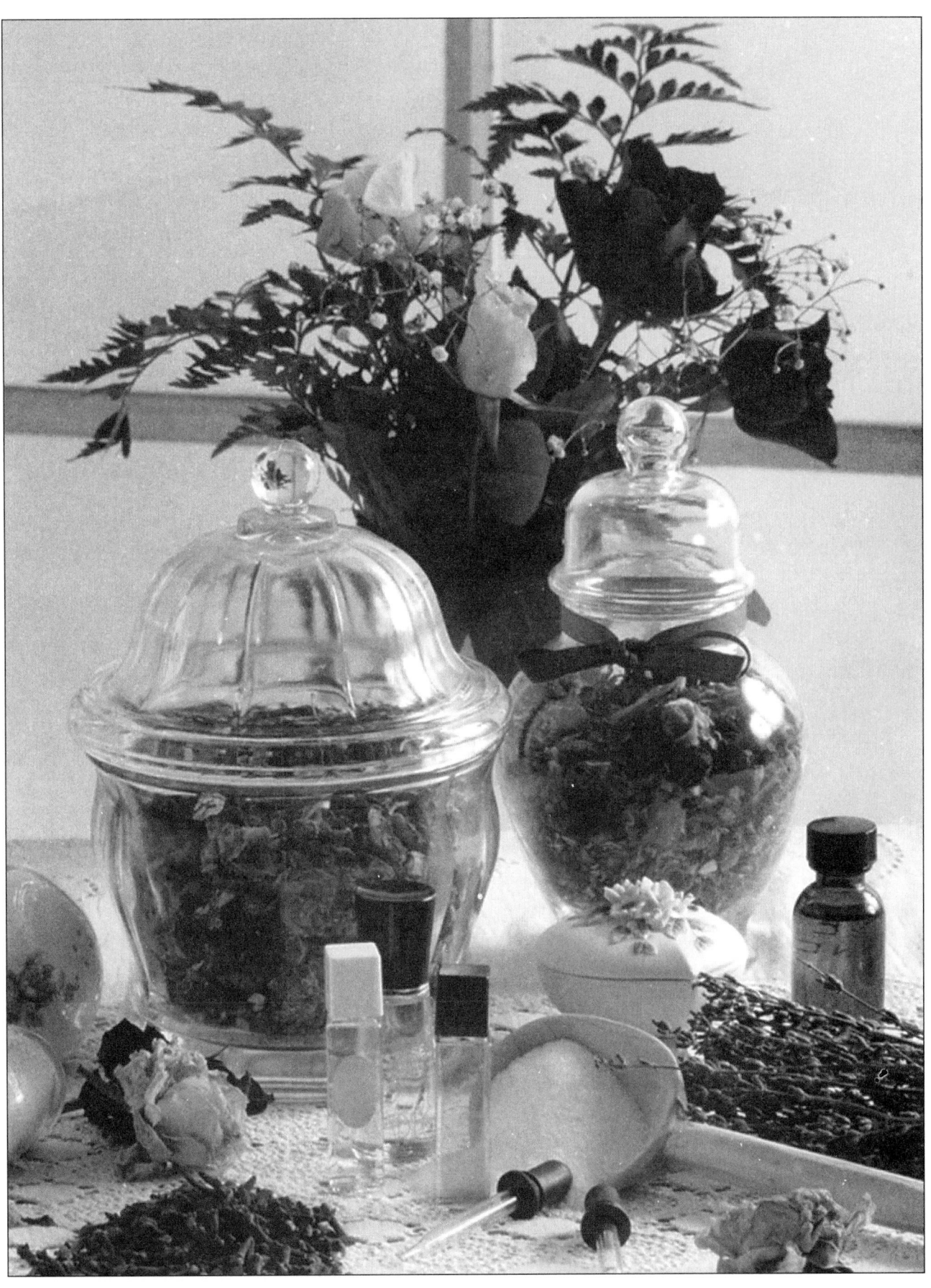

The Earth Shall Blossom

The following concoctions were selected from The Earth Shall Blossom, Shaker Herbs and Gardening *by Galen Beale and Mary Rose Boswell (The Countryman Press, Woodstock, Vt.). The authors worked at Shaker Village, Canterbury, N.H., where they studied 18th- and 19th-century documents and interviewed Shakers to compile a narrative of historical research, reminiscences and anecdotes.*

Rose Water

To collect ingredients for a potpourri, pick the petals in the morning after the dew is gone, but before noon.

Take of roses freshly gathered 6 pound, water 2 gallon. Distill off 1 gallon. Put this into glass bottles. Cover them with so many pieces of paper. Prickle full of holes & set them upon a table which is placed before a window where the sun will shine in upon them. After one month it will be fit for use. The first that blow out might be chilled down in some vessel until you get enough to distill it.

A simpler way to make rose water is to obtain rose soluble from a pharmacist. Dilute approximately 2½ teaspoons of the soluble with one pint of distilled water. A drop of red food coloring may be added if desired.

Rose Oil

Take a large jar and fill it [with] clean flowers of roses. Cover them with pure water and sit it in the sun in the day time and take in at night for seven days [or] when the oil will float on the top. Take this off with some cotton tied on a stick and squeeze in a phial and stop it up to close.

Use either pure spring water or rain water and remember to cover the crock if it looks like rain. The oil or attar looks like a yellowish oily scum and should be removed daily. Any herb oil can be extracted with these instructions.

To make your own cologne, try the following recipe. Collect a mixture of scented flowers and pack the blossoms in a jar and cover them with the pure ethyl or grain alcohol. Remove the blossoms and strain or squeeze the alcohol back into the jar, and fill the jar again with fresh blossoms. Repeat this procedure each day until the alcohol has reached the desired fragrance; then strain the cologne into bottles and seal tightly. To make the perfume last longer, add a small amount of fixative, such as ambergris, civet, or musk, in the general proportion of fifteen to one.

There are many flowers that can be used for a cologne, including the blossoms for the annual heliotrope, sweet alyssum, mignonette, petunia, sweet pea, phlox, and stock, as well as clematis, perennial dianthus, pe-

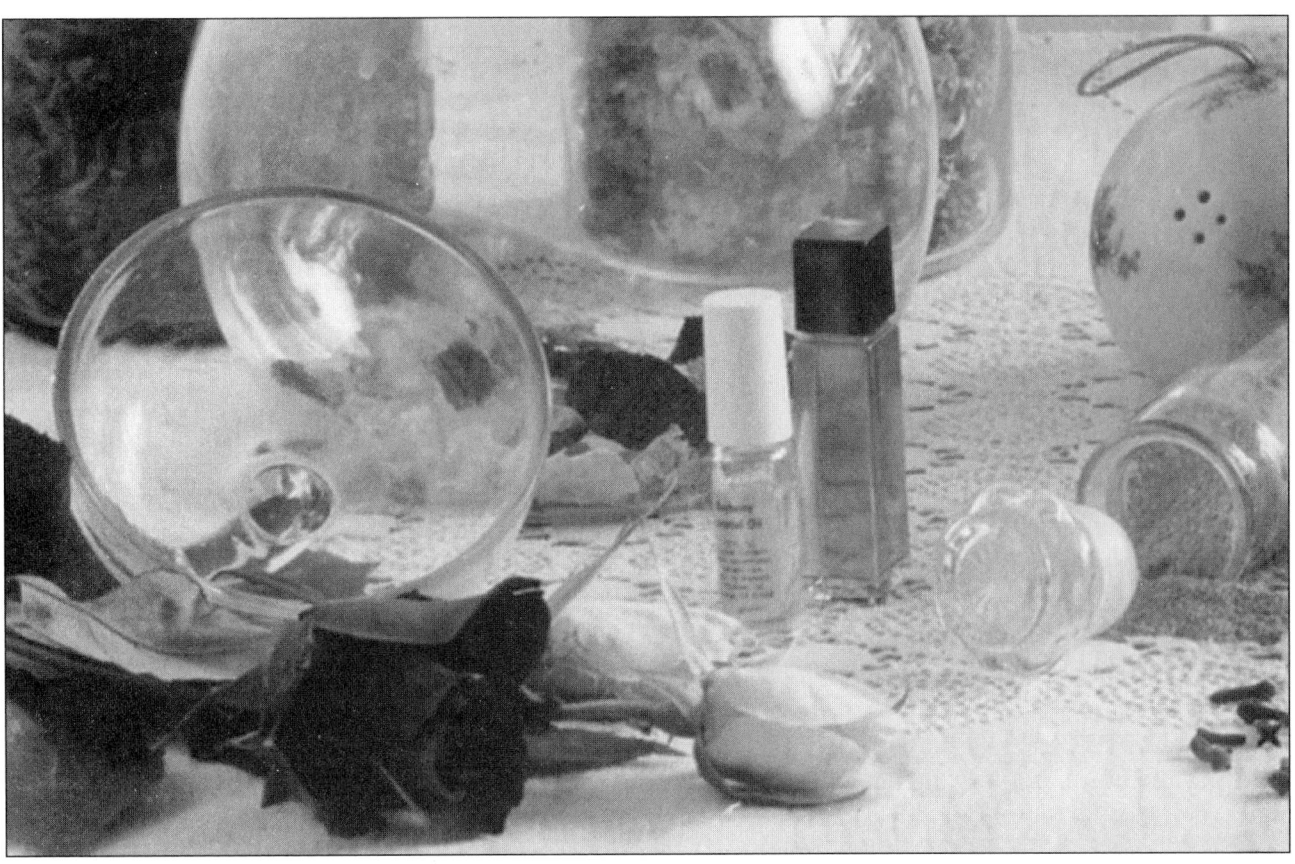

ony, salvia and sweet william.

Herbs such as lavender, rosemary, thyme, and lovage may be used as well as iris and daffodil. Try any flower you wish, but remember to keep a record of your experiments.

Rose Water and Witch Hazel Skin Tonic
Mix 2 parts rose water to 1 part witch hazel. The proportions of this refreshing skin tonic can be varied according to skin type.

Ointment of Rose Water
Take of Oil of almonds, two fluid ounces. Spermaceti, half an ounce, White wax one drachm. Melt the whole in a water bath, stirring it frequently; when melted add of Rosewater, two fluid drachms; And stir the mixture continually till it is cold.

The Shakers sold some of their herbal cosmetics to the World. The members claimed that "a few applications [of the Shaker Hair Restorer] will stop the falling out of the hair, and thus prevent baldness." A few years later they included the following quote in their Hair Restorer advertisement:

"It has been estimated," says the *New York Medical Record*, "that about one-half the adult men of American birth living in our cities are bald-headed." The estimate is not exaggerated, if it is applied to persons above the age of thirty, and it may be rather under the mark.

The probabilities point toward a race of hair-less Americans. The American nation is threatened with the catastrophe of a universal alopecia. From the visitors gallery of the Stock Exchange, for example, one views a mob of shining pates, belonging, as a rule, to rather young men.

The following is a recipe for a hair restorer used by the Groveland, New York, Shakers.

Hair Restorative
Put ½ pound pulv. Lobelia herb in a bottle, add to it equal parts of Whiskey, Brandy and Olive Oil. Bathe the head once a day, it will prevent the loss of hair & is said to restore it.

Potpourris Rose Jar
(using English Damask Roses)
Gather Rose petals in the morning, let them stand in a cool [place] toss them up lightly to dry, for

one hour then put them in layers, with salt sprinkled over each layer, in a large covered [jar]. A glass butter dish is a convenient receptial [sic]. Gather enough to make 4 pints to a quart according to the size of your jar. Stir then transfer to a glass fruit jar in the bottom of which you placed 2 ounces of allspice, coursely [sic] ground, 2 ounces of stick cinnamon broken coursely [sic].

When it is ready for the permanent jar, which may be as pretty as you please, those with double covers are the best, and very pretty ones in the blue and white Japanese ware, holding over 1 quart can be had for a few shillings. Now have ready 1 ounce each of cloves, allspice, cinnamon & Mace all ground not fine, 1 ounce Orris root bruised and shredded; 2 ounces of lavender flowers, and a small quantity of any other sweet scented flowers or herbs. Mix all together, and put into the jar in alternate layers with the Rose stock. Add a few drops of the Oil of Rose Geranium or Violet, and pour over the while add 1 gill [4 ounces] of good cologne. This will last for years though from time to time you may add a little lavender or Orange flower water or any nice perfume & some seasons, a few fresh rose petals. To use this open one hour every morning and then close.

To collect ingredients for a potpourri, pick the petals in the morning after the dew is gone, but before noon. Pick only as much as there is space to dry, for the petals need to be spread out in a single layer on a window screen or newspapers in a cool, dark place such as an attic or a closet. Whole buds and leaves may be selected; discard insects and soiled leaves and petals. Wait until the petals are chip dry, about 10 days to two weeks, stirring occasionally. Store the petals in a covered container, and they will keep indefinitely in a cool, dry place.

To make any potpourri, mix the petals and spices in the general proportions of one cup of dried petals to one teaspoon of fixative, one teaspoon of spices, and a drop or two of perfuming oil. Pack the mixture in closed containers and allow to age for six to eight weeks, stirring once in a while with a wooden spoon. Choose a pretty, clear, covered container to display the potpourri. Whole, dried blossoms may be affixed to the inside of a glass jar with dabs of beaten egg white. When they have dried on the jar sides, add the potpourri, and top with more whole dried blossoms.

Potpourri

　4　oz rose petals
　2　oz ground sandalwood
　1　oz whole cloves
　½　oz cinnamon
　½　oz allspice
　2　oz crushed orange peel
　1　oz powdered orris root
20　drops rose geranium oil
　6　drops oil of lavender
Age four to five weeks

Insect Repellants

Many herbs are effective moth repellants and include crushed bay leaves, feverfew, mint, pyrethrum, rosemary, southernwood, tansy, vetiver root, and wormwood. These are strong-scented herbs and are often blended with a dominating flower scent such as lavender.

For a simple moth repellant, collect and crush one quart of dried herbs of your choice, which may include lavender, peppermint, rosemary, santolina, southernwood, spearmint, tansy, thyme, woodruff, and wormwood. Add dried orange, lemon peel, and one teaspoon of either ground cloves, cinnamon or allspice.

Perfume & Preventative of Moths

Take of cloves, caraway seeds, nutmegs, mace, cinnamon, and Tonquin beans of each one ounce; Then add as much Florintine orris seed as will equal the other ingredients put together. Ground the whole well to powder, & then put it in little bags among your clothes.

Insect Repellant

The following is a modern insect repellant which you may also try: Combine equal amounts of fresh spearmint leaves, green onion tops, horseradish (roots and leaves), and cayenne pepper in 2 cups water. Mix in blender. Add 2 tablespoons of liquid detergent. Keep in refrigerator. ◆

Sheep Nanny Tea

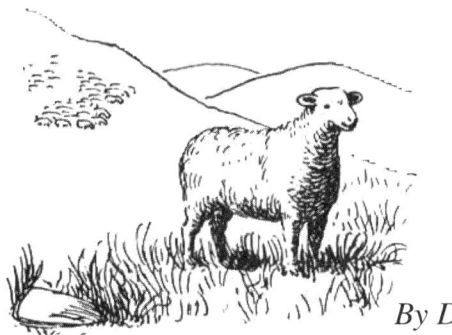

By Dale Morrison

I think that child's coming down with the measles," Grandma Laura said.

"Heaven forbid!" Mama shook her head so hard that the combs fell out of her long, blond hair. "She's just got over the whooping cough!"

"What does that have to do with the price of eggs in China?" Grandma snapped her store-bought teeth together and set her mouth above her square chin in that thin pink line that had inspired Senator Downey's famous remark, "Ira Morrison's wife is the stubbornest female in southwestern Pennsylvania!"

The year was 1921; we were Democrats; I was 8 years old. Mama and her mother-in-law were at it again. They were both schoolteachers and aggravatingly aggressive women, Grandma having fought for women's rights and Mama having helped spearhead the Prohibition movement. Grandma had a rowdy sense of humor while Mama was the sobersides of the family.

As befitted the bone of contention, I retreated behind the Kalamazoo stove. I itched all over. The itch was so universal that it was hopelessly unscratchable. I squirmed helplessly in my long underwear. I felt swollen and boilish, as though my shoe tops were cutting into my flesh.

At that time of year—early January—I hated every garment I wore. This condition persisted from the first of November until the middle of March, for little girls were not dressed beautifully in those days. The keynotes of apparel were serviceability, warmth and economy. We went to school clad in bulky dark blues and browns and wadded our union-suited legs into lumpy, dun-colored stockings held up by supporters.

Most of us had blisters on our heels. Our feet were encased in clumsy, unyielding shoes which laced above the ankle. Colorful clothing, except toboggan caps and occasionally mittens, was frowned upon as a reflection of the mother's frivolity.

I was miserably hot inside and my pale, square-cut bangs clung damply to my forehead. Yet I longed to crawl inside the oven, because no matter how closely I hugged the stove, it gave me no comfort.

"Open your mouth," Mama ordered, dragging me forth bodily. She peered down my throat. "Look, Grandma," she commanded. "No strawberry tongue."

Grandma pushed her spectacles up on her nose. She gazed long and learnedly into my innards. "Pshaw, Bessie," she snorted. "That means nothing. As you well know, the measles are going around now, and this child seems to have your unhappy faculty of picking up every germ that she comes in contact with."

Grandma brushed back my bangs and gazed into my eyes. "Her forehead is hotter than the hinges of Hades. I do declare, you'd better take her temperature."

Mama swore at Grandma with her eyes as only a lady could in those days, and dutifully poked the thermometer under my parched tongue. "Shut your mouth, keep quiet and don't talk," she ordered, although I hadn't said a word.

Holding the thermometer in place with the tip of my forefinger, I slithered carefully into the wicker rocking chair beside the water tank. Mama and Grandma silently began to set the table. Meals were always on time in that household, and even though Mama fiercely resented living with her in-laws, it was a big house and its men were hearty eaters and good providers.

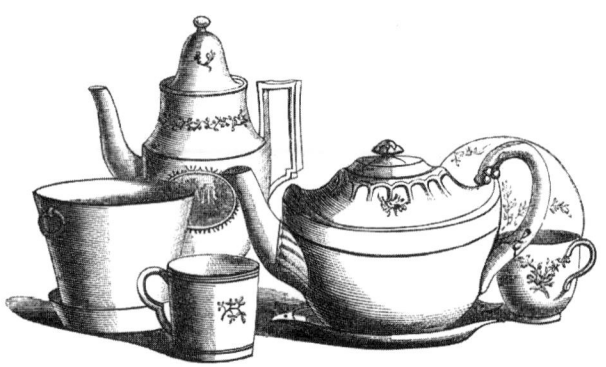

I rocked quietly, thermometer in my mouth, concentrating hard: *No measles, no measles. Please, Lord—and everybody—no measles.* There, dwarfed by the shadows in that huge kitchen, I remained forgotten until Papa came roaring in in a plume of cold, stamping the snow from his boots.

"What's the matter with you, towhead?" Papa shouted.

"Oh," exclaimed Mama, "I almost forgot!" She hastily yanked the thermometer out of my mouth and held it under the light. "Ninety-nine even," she announced triumphantly. "Hardly anything at all. I told you there was nothing to be alarmed about."

"Nevertheless, she is running a slight temperature," Grandma persisted. "Feed her lightly and put her to bed right after supper."

I fed lightly indeed, for my appetite had fled with the waning daylight. I felt old—I thought, *older than Grandma looks; older than Grandpa.*

I sat next to Grandpa at the table. Ira Morrison, with his wavy, white hair, iron-gray Vandyke and twinkly blue eyes, was a veritable saint of a man, given to 20-minute prayers at the table. However, he owned a vast profusion of good humor which made his official visits as the county superintendent a gala occasion at any school in our district.

"What's the matter with my bright little girl tonight?" he boomed. "You're just pecking at your plate like a chickabiddy."

"I don't feel so good," I whispered, aware that I had just become the focus of four pairs of eyes which were the brains of Washington Township. Life with the senior Morrisons was like a continual visit to the principal's office for one small third-grader. To top that off, half the kids at school distrusted me on sight because all of my relatives were in the teaching profession.

"She's coming down with the measles," Grandma said, giving Mama a cool stare and passing the lima beans to Papa.

"Don't say that, Grandma," Mama spunked, "just because the measles are going around."

"You'll have to keep her home if she's broken out by morning," Grandpa said, and Mama turned pale.

I knew what Mama feared. She hated—simply loathed—the idea of another quarantine. I had already kept her indoors with my bouts of chicken pox and whooping cough.

"Bessie doesn't want to admit the possibility of having to give up more of her cherished club meetings," Grandma snorted. "After all, whether she likes it or not, she is the child's mother."

Mama bit her lip and lowered her full eyelids. Miserably I felt her resentment and helplessness, brought up in our rigid community tradition that one did not sass one's elders no matter *what* they said. Grandma, who had served her own sentence under an autocratic mother-in-law, enjoyed needling Mama above all other household games.

Then Papa, gesturing as if struck with a thought, bumbled to the rescue, a gambit known in our clan as "changing the subject." "Say, Mother," he chuckled, "remember the old home remedy you threatened me with when I was a kid?"

Grandma grinned. "Maybe we'll have to give this child a little dose."

Grandpa laughed and Mama sniffed.

"A dose of what?" I quavered. My voice sounded thin and lost. Visions of paregoric and castor oil flashed through my mind. Every time I sneezed or sighed, somebody was coming at me with a spoonful of nasty-tasting medicine.

"Never mind," Grandma said. "Eat your pudding and ask me after we leave the table."

Due to my delicate condition, I was excused from drying the dishes, and sought the companionable comfort of my friend, the big stove. I had no intention of asking Grandma what the dose was.

When Papa and Grandpa came in from bedding down the stock, Papa said, "Has anybody brewed the sheep nanny tea?"

Mama said, "Oh, hush, Jack!"

Grandma turned to me, a gleam in her eye. "Ollie, did you know that when I was a youngster, folks made youngsters drink sheep nanny tea to bring out the measles?"

"Sure enough," Grandpa added. "It was a common thing in our day."

I choked at the thought. I knew what sheep nannies were. Spacing my words very carefully, I asked, "What was sheep nanny tea made of?"

Everybody guffawed at that—even Mama. Grandpa shook with merriment, Papa fairly rolled on the floor, and Grandma laughed till she cried. "Sheep nannies," she said finally, wiping her eyes with the corner of her blue gingham apron.

"Dried, of course, not fresh," Grandpa explained.

"Didn't it make them sick?" I asked, stalling for time, for the horrible thought struck me. I had been through scenes like this before—talk of laxatives always led to castor oil, and discussion of parasites led inevitably to vermifuge. I was becoming convinced that I would end up imbibing sheep nanny tea.

Visions of sheep nannies floated before my eyes, rich fruit of the pasture clustered in random heaps like lavish handfuls of plump raisins. Such earthy leavings as modern children call "smart pills"—these were sheep nannies.

"There may be something to the theory after all," Papa boomed jovially. "Heaven only knows what wonders science may reveal." Papa was a pioneer in organic chemistry which I only vaguely understood as a study of how natural things are put together.

"The sheep, I would have you know, is one of the cleanest of animals," Grandma said staunchly, "a strict and selective vegetarian." I could picture her hovering over the stove like an old witch at midnight, brewing a heady potful of sheep nanny tea.

"Ergo," chuckled Grandpa, "sheep nannies may well be composed of the finest herbs, predigested and internally refined."

At this point, tears began to sting my eyes. My grown-ups were sometimes overwhelming.

"Hush your nonsense," Mama cried. "The child is sniffling. See what I told you—she just has a touch of cold." And, thoroughly exasperated, she took me by the arm. "Here, Ollie, you get off to bed with a couple of hot bricks to your feet."

"Yes, Mama," I said, almost tripping her up in my eagerness to get upstairs. This was unusual, for I really hated going up to bed. But those visions of a mysterious, dark brown potion expedited my departure.

"I still say she's getting the measles," Grandma called after as we climbed the stairs.

Why didn't they call the doctor? In our community in 1921, nobody called the doctor for children's diseases. Minor epidemics of these were considered to be the normal heritage of childhood, and it was better to have them and get over them than to sit around and wonder when they would strike. All mothers and grandmothers were supposed to be fully endowed by the simple fact of parenthood with the ability to diagnose and deal with these minor ailments.

After one "broke out" with measles or chicken pox, or when mumps became visible, a doctor might put in a brief appearance, give a couple of pills and some laughing advice and, if he were the local health officer, tack up a quarantine sign. Doctors were luxuries reserved for grown-up illnesses, broken bones, "serious" epidemics and bringing babies in their black bags. Doctors were also employed to chop out tonsils and adenoids, as I knew only too well.

I realized, as I padded off to bed, that I was in a very serious spot. I would have to be either better or worse by morning; no halfway measures were permitted. A school-age child was either sick or well. If you were not sick you were well, and off to school you went. There was no staying home to find out. Coddling the young was considered slightly sinful, and family honor was measured by attendance record.

"A dose of what?" I quavered. Every time I sneezed or sighed, somebody was coming at me with a spoonful of nasty-tasting medicine.

Mama tucked me in with hot bricks and even allowed me the unheard-of luxury of leaving a low fire in my room. "Mind you, stay covered up," she admonished, and tiptoed out, leaving me to watch the pink and lavender flickerings against the ceiling from the gas burner.

As I lay there, I could hear night sounds from the farm outside. What oppressed me particularly was the distant *baa*-ing of sheep. I imagined the wooly creatures nannying as they bleated. I had a nasty taste in my mouth, and I dropped off to sleep pretending that wolves were chasing all the sheep into the river. Somehow in my dreams the good guys got mixed up with the bad, and I woke shrieking just as a sheep with huge slavering jaws was about to swallow me whole.

As soon as I sat up in bed I knew I had pulled an awful boner. The door opened, the light was turned on, and the whole crew came pounding in—Grandpa in his long flannel night rail, Papa in his shabby bathrobe, Mama and Grandma, plaits flying, still bundling themselves into their flowered wrappers.

"Ollie, Ollie," Mama cried, "you'll raise the whole countryside!"

"My goodness, Bessie," exclaimed Grandma, "the child's having a nightmare."

"I feel awful," I managed to say, clutching dramatically at my throat which did feel horribly sticky and raw.

Then Grandpa uttered a magnificent "Hist!" and beckoned Papa outside for a conference while Mama and Grandma, clucking like two hens, peered down my throat with a flashlight. Then Grandpa came tiptoeing back and tapped Grandma on the shoulder. She scurried away. I could hear the three of them whispering while Mama, looking daggers at the door, plumped up my pillows. In a few moments Grandma stuck her head into the room and intoned, "Bessie, come!"

Mama muttered something and joined the conference. I heard them all troop downstairs, shutting the doors all the way down to the kitchen. Distinctly I heard laughter and scolding and the clatter of pans. Thoroughly alarmed, I shook off the heavy quilts and tried to climb out of bed.

It was my intent to creep downstairs and listen, but suddenly they were all back like a circus parade. Grandma was carrying a huge, steaming cup. I ducked under the covers but Papa dragged me out. He held one hand under my chin. "Drink it down," Grandma ordered, while Mama hopped helplessly from one foot to the other and wrung her hands.

A pungent odor rose from the cup. The liquid was a sickening deep amber and its vapor made my eyes smart. I tried to push it away, but Grandpa held my hands. "It's good for you," he said gruffly but kindly. "Don't think about it—just drink it down fast."

It was years before I found out what had been in that cup. My family, fanatics that they were, had conspired to give me a far worse thing than sheep nanny tea. They had contrived a home remedy guaranteed to cure the ills of man and beast, namely a toddy of whiskey, lemon juice, hot water and brown sugar. It was the presence of "medicinal" alcohol which sealed their lips. Two WCTU members in good standing and two ardent Prohibitionists could hardly let it be known that they were feeding their offspring "devil's brew." It was, I suppose, proof of their great concern that they made the sacrifice and said nothing.

The liquid stung my throat. I gulped and gagged, but swallowed. I *had* to swallow;

Grandma was holding my nose. The stuff went down like swill and I died a thousand deaths of humiliation. I finally managed to kick my legs free and knock the cup out of Grandma's hand. I fought them, screaming, "I hate you! I hate you! You made me drink poo-poos!" And, retching violently, I waggled off to the bathroom and heaved into the basin.

I heard Mama say, "Serves you right."

Papa said, "I'd spank her if she weren't sick."

Grandpa and Grandma seemed to be holding each other up, shaking with helpless laughter. Right-eously indignant, I pranced back to bed, glaring my defiance. "If you make me drink any more sheep nanny tea, I'll throw up all over you," I declared. "Now go away and turn off the light."

For the first and last time in my young life, I gave the orders. Like whipped dogs they slunk away. But Grandma, of course, had to have the last word. She popped her head back in the door and hissed, "If you're not broke out by morning, I *will* give you sheep nanny tea."

I went to sleep thinking, *Please Lord— measles! Cross out that other prayer. Just give me the measles and I'll be a good girl.*

When I awoke it was daylight. I crept out of bed and looked in the big mirror over the bureau. I was covered with red spots. I was peppered, but suddenly I felt good. I went pounding down the stairs and bounced into the kitchen. There they all stood, cups in their

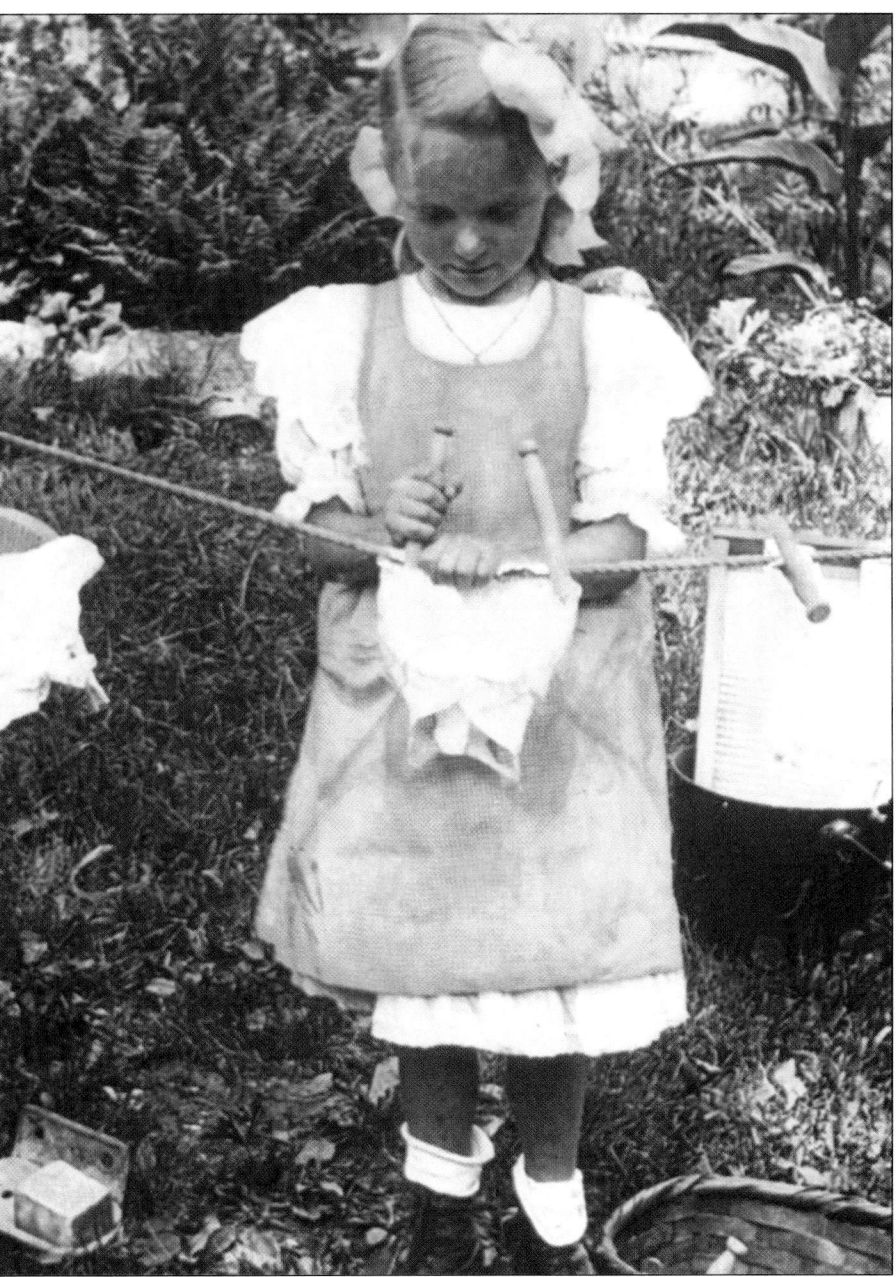

hands. "Whee!" I yelped. "Look at me! I've got measles!"

"First time I ever saw a youngster happy over measles," Grandpa said. Papa slapped his leg with fiendish glee.

"No sheep nanny tea?" I asked. "I won't have to drink any more sheep nanny tea, will I?"

"No," said Mama. "No sheep nanny tea." She looked at Grandma.

"I guess the child just had to break out—or else," Grandma said. And for once Grandma and Mama laughed together over their private joke. ◆

Beauty by the Season

By Josephine Bailey

Mother had a green thumb and she used it to the best of her ability. She grew all sorts of vegetables, as well as herbs to season the delicious food she cooked, but it was her flower garden which gave us practical beauty secrets which we have used throughout our lives.

In the old days we didn't have the fancy beauty preparations we have today. But Mother had a beauty treatment for any need. Olive oil and even chicken fat were used extensively as a hair conditioner and lubricant for dry skin. Top-milk and cream were standard purifiers and moisturizers for a beautiful complexion.

Vinegar, lemon and cucumber were used as astringents. We rubbed them on our faces, giving ourselves facial massages which stimulated the skin. Sterilized earth mixed with water substituted for a mud pack.

In spring when flowers were abundant, roses played a special role in our daily beauty routine. Sitting in the garden with friends, we'd pluck petals and rub our cheeks with them. Mother would laughingly remark, "Now you have cheeks as pink as a rose."

Rose petals distilled in hot water made a fragrant preparation for the bath or to use as the base for perfume. At the end of June when strawberries were in season, we'd rub the ripe berries on our faces. Today there is a strawberry facial

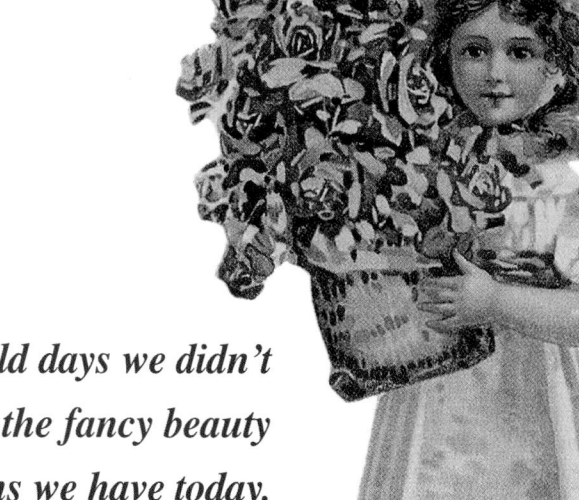

In the old days we didn't have the fancy beauty preparations we have today. But Mother had a beauty treatment for any need.

cream on the market!

A cotton pad dipped in mint tea and placed on closed eyelids was a great reliever for tired eyes.

We made a soothing skin ointment from balsam leaves and flowers. We dried other flowers and used them throughout the year. We sewed lavender into aromatic sachets for our bureau drawers and closets. On autumn evenings, we were busy tying crushed dried flowers into small net bags to be used as Christmas gifts.

In the summer, Mama constantly worried about our hair and bodies being exposed to the hot sun. We had to protect ourselves by wearing wide-brimmed hats. We rubbed Vaseline or olive oil onto our skin after being out in the sun. After an afternoon at the beach, a baking soda bath was a must to rinse off the saltwater and cool our sunburned skin. At the end of the vacation season we used lemon or cucumber juice to bleach out what was left of our summer sunburn. There were no commercial suntan lotions in those days—but we managed on our own using nature's remedies.

Autumn was windy and rainy. Raining? Put

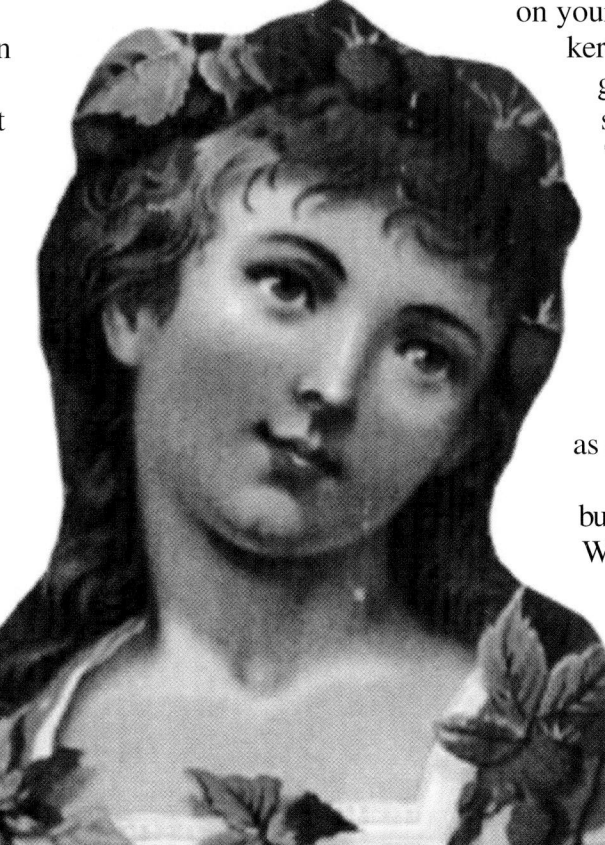

Today there are hundreds of different beauty preparations. But I still remember Mother's advice and use rose, lemon, cucumber and natural cream in my daily beauty routine.

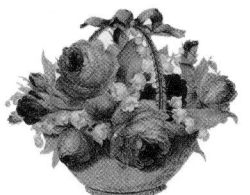

on your raincoat, rubbers, and a kerchief over your head—and go take a walk. This was sound advice from Mama. The wind whipped our faces; the rain cleansed our clogged pores, leaving us with rosy complexions. Chapped hands and faces were treated with cream, leaving our skin as smooth as silk.

Winter was a problem, but Mother knew how to cope. We applied a mask of Vaseline to our hands and faces as a shield against the bitter winter wind. It was not beyond Mama's reason to let us rub snow on our faces to stimulate circulation. After a snowy frolic, we'd sit by the fire and apply cream to our faces. In these days of homogenized milk we miss the cream which rose to the top of the milk bottle! It was one of the best skin softeners, and I'm sure it is used in many commercial formulas today.

Today there are hundreds of different beauty preparations. But I still remember Mother's advice and use rose, lemon, cucumber and natural cream in my daily beauty routine.

Although I am now of retirement age, I am proud to say that, like Mother's face in her 80s, mine does not show a single wrinkle! ◆

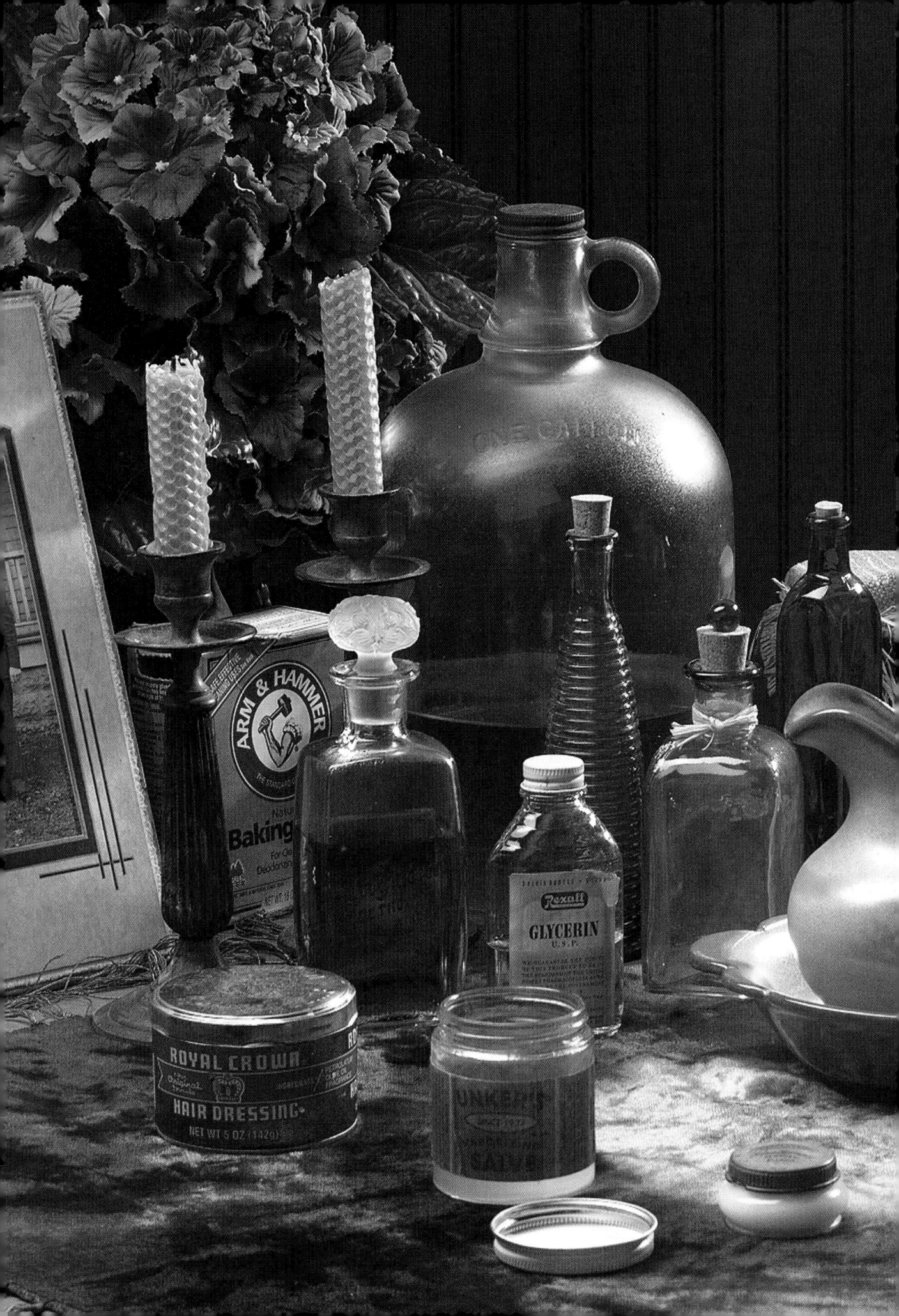

Chapter 4

MIRACLES OR MYTHS?

There is a part of medicine and doctoring that was left behind when our health system moved from home remedies and country doctors to specialists and huge hospitals. Cold science can't explain some things, so it dismisses that which cannot be examined in the laboratory.

How many of us had a parent, uncle or neighbor who could remove warts? My wife's Grandpa Barnes could—and she is a living witness to his abilities. When she was a little girl, Grandpa did his magic and her unsightly warts disappeared in a few days. To this day she wishes she had asked him how he did it.

What about blood stoppers, faith healers and the mysterious madstone that cured rabies? They're not talked about much today in our modern world, but were clearly the cures of choice when there was nowhere else to turn. Enjoy these stories of home-cure miracles both small and great.

—Ken Tate

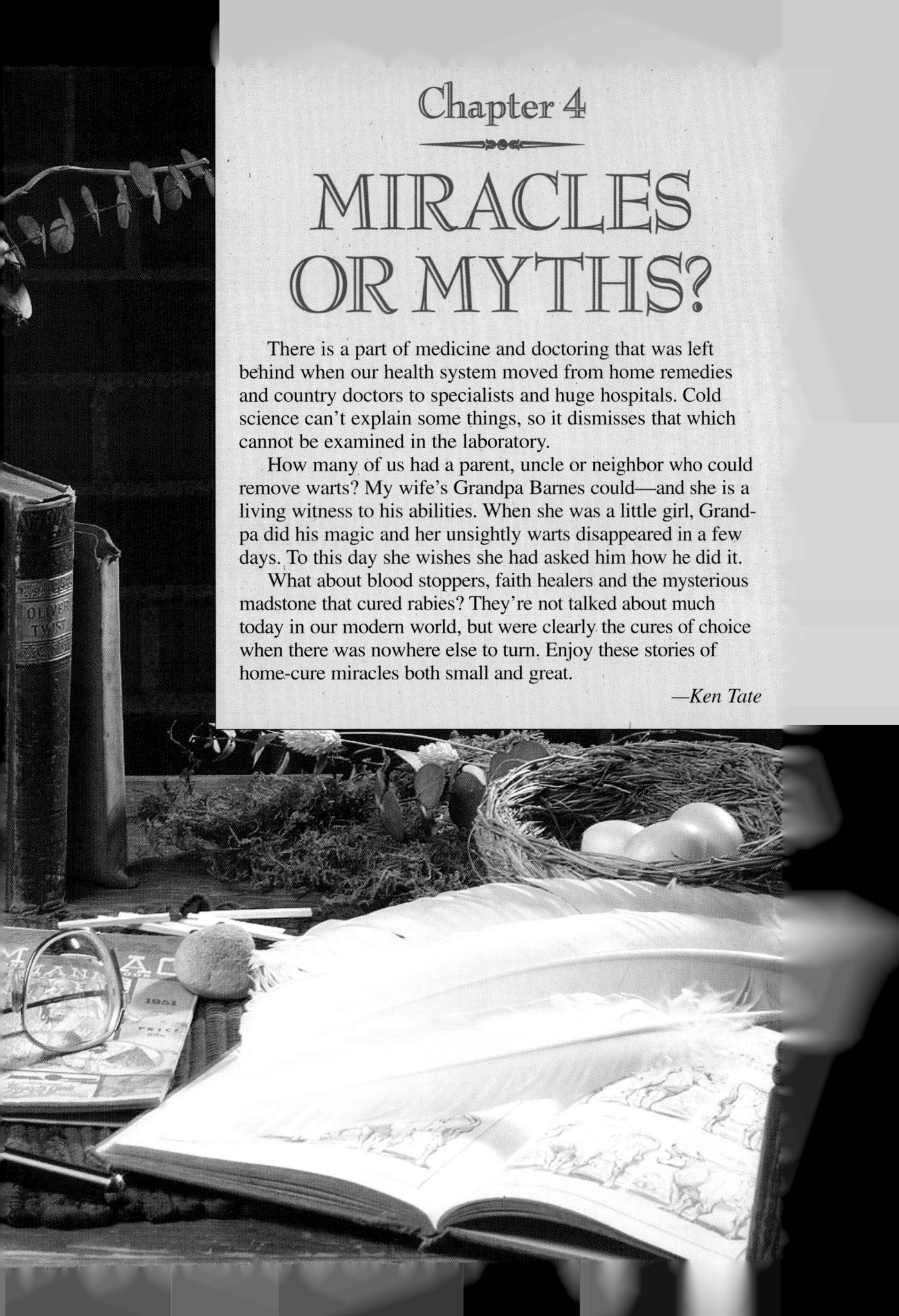

Myth or Miracle?

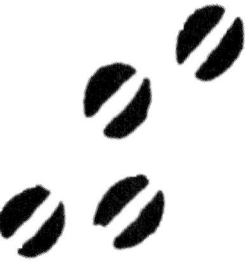

DEER TRACKS

By Leta Fulmer

They felt almost warm against the moist skin of my palms, these talismans of the past, and I felt a sense of awe and mystery which perhaps bordered on the ridiculous in a sensible middle-age woman. But then, this *was* the Nelson Madstone, whose mystic power purportedly had been the only hope for those bitten by a rabid animal in the 1800s.

As a child I had listened in rapt and shivering fear as Mom had told me of dogs which used to roam the streets and farmlands, frothing at the mouth, ready to snap repeatedly at anything in their path. There were no rabies shots then, no cure or protection from the horrible death that was almost a certainty if one were infected. No fairy story ever held me more spellbound than Mom's description of people rushing prayerfully toward the madstone to enlist its curative powers.

Until recently, I hadn't dreamed that it still existed. Now, thanks to the Savannah (Mo.) Historical Society, I could actually touch this almost-forgotten wonder. I leaned closer to inspect them.

Originally in one piece, now there were two, each about the size of a thin nickel. Like small bits of gravel held together with shellac, they were encircled by silver bands. Their many years of service had indeed taken their toll.

I listened, entranced, as the owner began his speech.

It was 1844. There had been a killing. With the help of John and James Nelson, the murderer managed to escape, vowing to return and repay the twins for their help.

Can you imagine their chagrin when he returned two years later from the East Indies and presented their reward? No gold, nor sparkling jewels—only an odd-looking stone taken from the heart of a male deer. Supposedly it possessed the power to cure the lethal bite of a mad dog.

They must have thought he considered them gullible beyond belief, but in those days, when there was no protection from the bite of a rabid animal, what was to be lost in trying? And in the trying, that small stone became famous in our area and far beyond. It was the only straw to cling to when the fearful cry "Mad dog!" was heard.

The Nelson boys sawed the stone in half when they separated,

Between 1881 and 1931, more than 2,000 patients were treated with the Nelson Madstone.

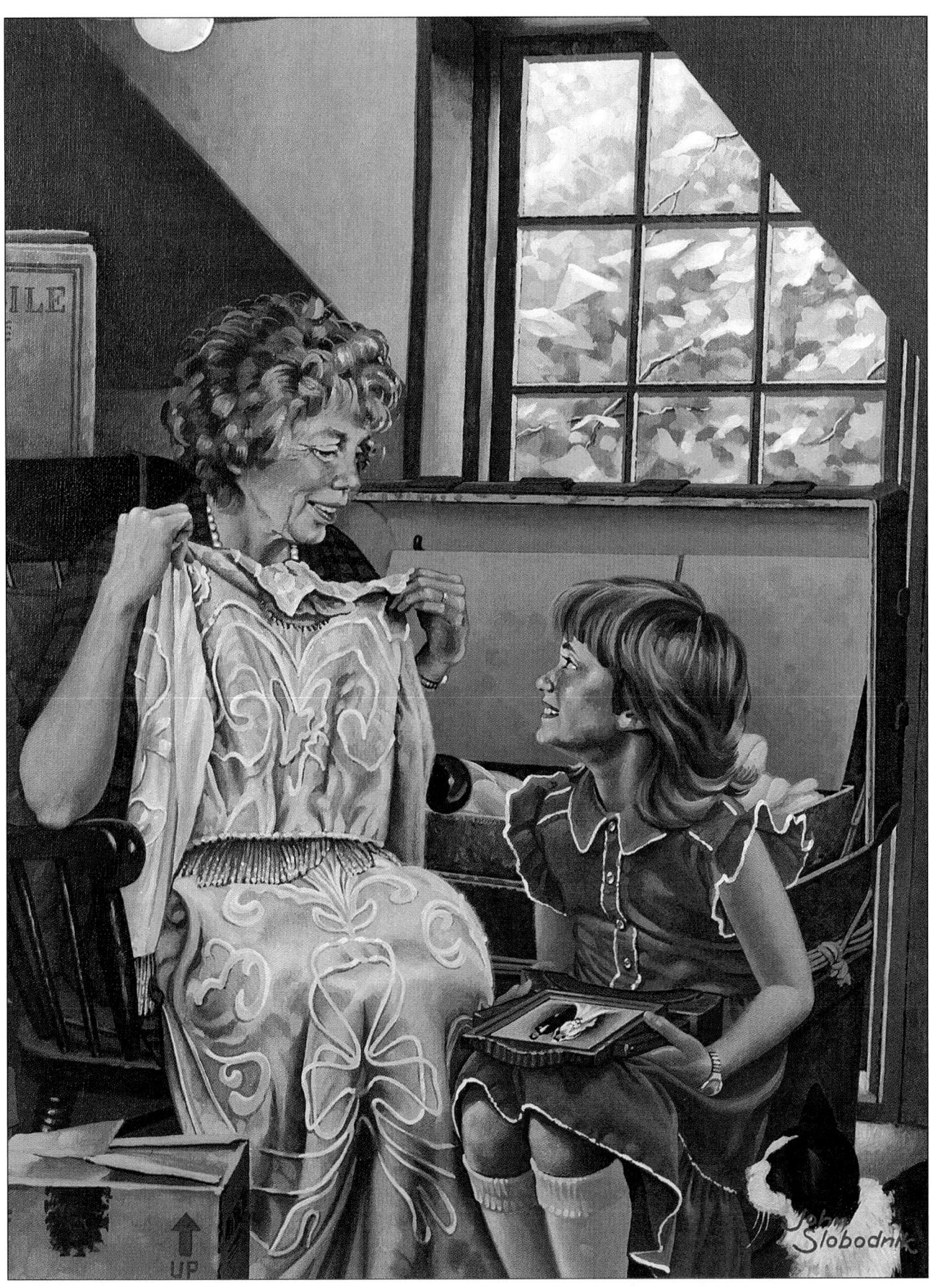

though James later returned his piece to John, who kept them until he died in 1897. John's daughter, Armede Humber, inherited the stone and continued the records that dated from 1881 to 1931 when rabies were brought under medical control. During that time more than 2,000 patients were treated, many coming from faraway communities, even distant states. During those years when the stones were in constant use, both halves burst. For a time the pieces were held together with string; later they were secured with the silver bands.

As the speaker continued, I could almost envision the little girl who'd been attacked by a strange dog as she reached out to stroke his head. I could imagine her frantic father's grief as he urged the horses to greater speed, their buggy jogging crazily along the twisting road toward Savannah—and the Nelson Madstone. I could picture the fear in the mother's face, and imagine her fervent prayers as she cradled the injured child in her arms. Certainly the flickering lamplight at their destination must have shown like a beacon through the dark, and in the modest home, the little girl was made ready for treatment.

A sterile needle drew blood from the wound which was then bathed in a solution of vinegar and salt. The stone itself was soaked in warm milk, then blown dry.

For several hours the stone clung tightly to the wound, attesting to the presence of the poison there. When it fell off of its own accord, it was cleansed in milk which slowly turned a greenish hue.

That little girl lived to thrill her grandchildren with her story, as did many others

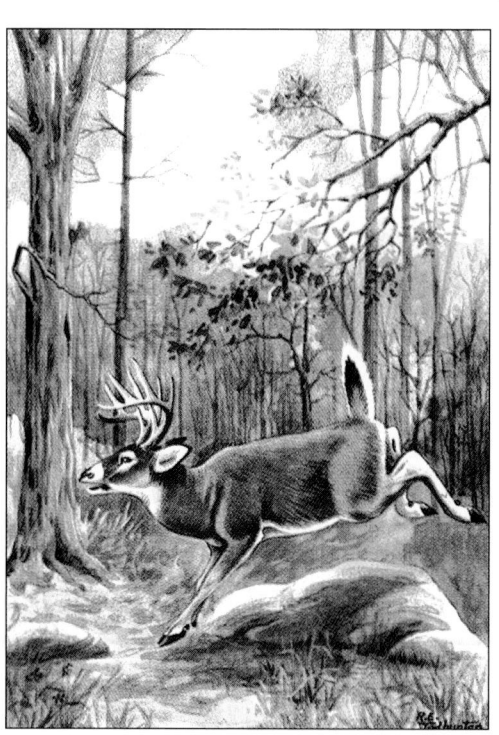

As their reward, they received no gold, nor sparkling jewels—only an odd-looking stone taken from the heart of a male deer.

who made similar trips in fear and trepidation. And the price? Five dollars if the stone did not stick; $25 if the madstone adhered to the wound and worked its magic power.

The Nelson Madstone is idle now, an almost-forgotten bit of yesteryear. It is the property of Mr. and Mrs. Ralph Metcalf of St. Joseph, Mo. At the historical meeting I leafed through the yellowed scrapbook of newspaper clippings. I searched through the small notebook filled with names and addresses, details of visits and cures, and I held the stones again, almost loath to see them tucked into the old-fashioned coin purse in which they've been kept for so many years. The antique saucer which held them during the soaking process is a treasure in itself, still unchipped after many years of service.

As I tried to capture the images of these items on film, I felt I was snaring a bit of history for my very own—a fairy tale pulled from the past into the present. In this day of scientific wonders, this story may sound a little like native incantations or black magic, I know, but heart transplants still seem like Dr. Frankenstein to me, and acupuncture certainly has all the earmarks of voodoo. With a chuckle, I can't help but wonder how John Nelson would accept the fact of man walking on the moon!

Which is it? Fact or fantasy? Myth or miracle? Take your pick; I realize now that I made my choice long ago with the blind faith of a child. Seeing the Nelson Madstone has only strengthened my belief, for after all, what is life itself but a mystery to ponder and a miracle to believe in? ◆

The Madstone

By Paul G. Brewster

In earlier days—and even into the present century in some sections of the country—doctors were few and far between. This fact, along with the poor communication systems and bad roads, made it necessary for the sick and injured to be treated with remedies available in the area. Most of these came from plants—fennel, hartshorn, sassafras, rhubarb, arrowroot, plantain, elder, dandelion, mullein and jewelweed, to name a few.

But such remedies were ineffective against some attacks on health and life. When someone was stung by a poisonous insect, bitten by a snake, or by a rabid fox or dog, the only sure antidote was the madstone.

In earlier days, when someone was stung by a poisonous insect, bitten by a snake, or by a rabid fox or dog, the only sure antidote was the madstone.

In some parts of the world, the stone appears in the stomach or entrails of monkeys, goats, porcupines or other animals; in the United States, it is said to be found only in the stomach of an albino deer. Why the deer must be albino has never been explained.

The stone is applied directly to the wound. It adheres tightly and, being porous, sucks up the poison. Eventually it loosens its grip and falls off. Then it is immersed in a vessel of sweet milk, which takes on a greenish color. The stone is applied a second time and again put into the milk after it has dropped off. The process is repeated until the stone will no longer adhere to the wound, or until the milk ceases to turn green. In one case, treatment continued for 13 hours!

Madstones were cherished possessions in the United States and in England, from whence many were brought to this country in Colonial times. They were handed down from father to son, and rarely—if ever—sold. The fortunate possessor was glad to permit others to use it, and always without charge, as it was believed that charging for such service would make the madstone useless thereafter.

Among noted persons who possessed madstones were the French monarch Charles IX, Sir Walter Raleigh, Gov. Endicott of Massachusetts and Gov. Winthrop of Connecticut.

Despite advances in medicine, belief in the power of a madstone has persisted in some areas of the United States. But though it was once known and used nationwide, it is now remembered only in relatively isolated areas—portions of the Ozarks, the Cumberland Mountains, the Great Smokies, and some sections of Kentucky and West Virginia.

Now treasured more as heirlooms than as antidotes, a number of madstones still exist. I know of three in Kentucky and three more in Tennessee. The owner of one of these was offered—and refused—$2,000 for it. ◆

Nita and the Stone

By J.B. Cearley

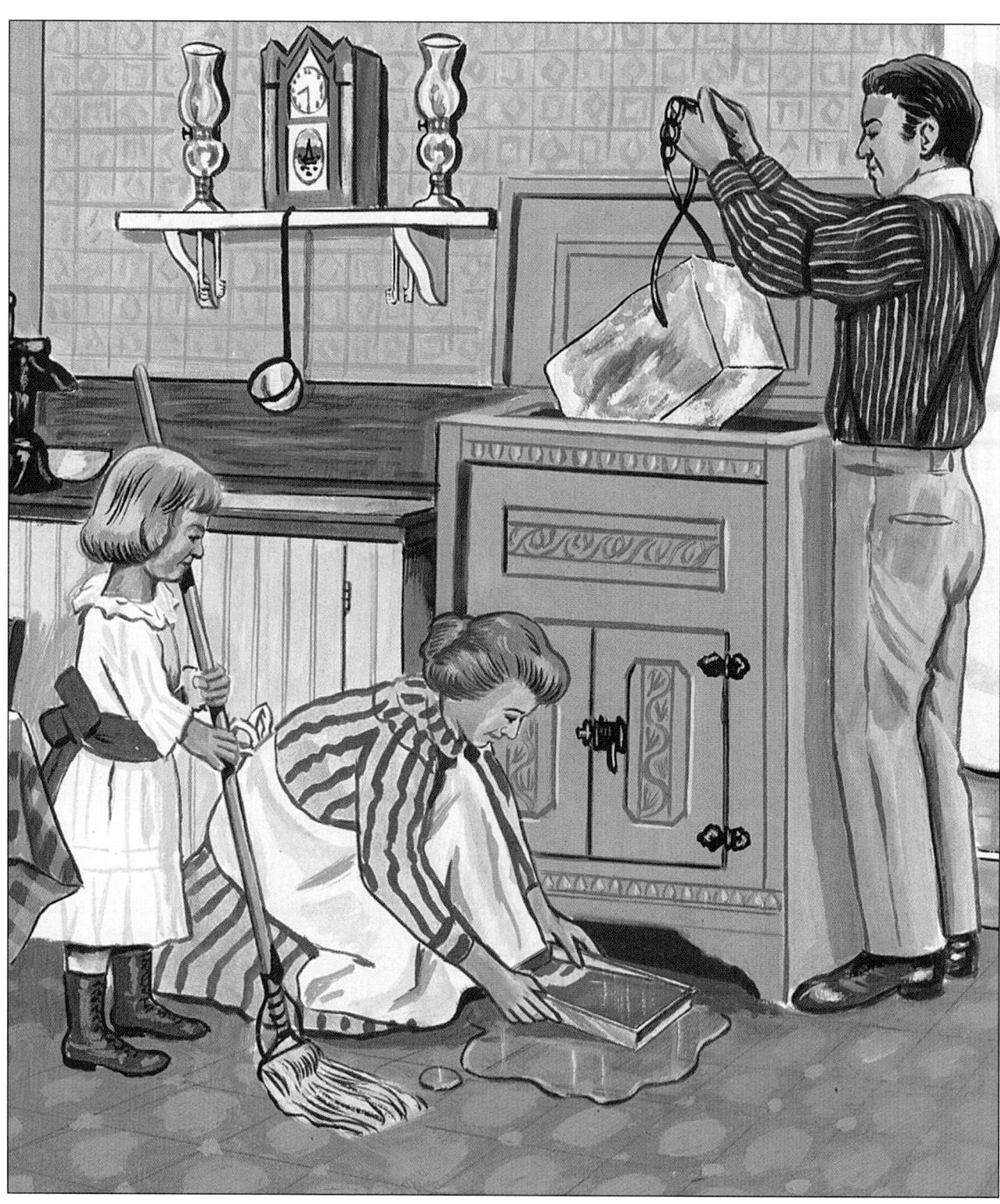

Fortunately, the blistering heat and dry weather had hit Central Texas in late August. Most of the crops were made and were being gathered. The corn crop was harvested, and people were picking cotton on the great blackland farms.

The temperature hovered at 105 degrees just before sundown. Ellen Carson spoke to her husband while they were eating supper. "I just do not see how we can sleep in the house tonight. It's almost like an oven in here."

Tim Carson glanced around the small house. They were cooped up in a sweatbox like canned sardines. He glanced at 4-year-old Nita who was playing with her food. "Eat your supper, honey," he coaxed.

"Too hot," the child replied. "I'm not very hungry."

Tim watched her nibble at the red, ripe tomato from their garden. Nita paused and sipped from her glass of cool milk. Ellen had kept the milk in a small container in the cooler Tim had made in the kitchen window. Ellen poured fresh water from the dug well over cloths hanging above and around the milk jars. The little breeze that blew in from the west helped create an evaporative air-conditioner effect to keep the milk cool.

Ellen stopped to wipe her forehead with a damp cloth. "It's just too hot. I wish we had electric power in the country so we could have a fan. That would be a help in this beastly weather."

"Fall will come soon and cool us off," Tim said hopefully. "This heat can't last forever."

"How can we sleep on those hot beds tonight?"

"Well, how about sleeping on the porch? That'll be the coolest place we can find about dusk."

Ellen thought for a moment. "Yes, that would be nice. We can move the mattresses. It's just too hot for little Nita."

So it was that the Carson family began sleeping on the big porch of their three-room home that August in 1922. They found it to be hot, but some better than the heat-infested house. When a breeze blew, they got the full benefit of the air current.

Sometime during the midnight hours of their fourth night on the porch, Ellen was awakened by a piercing scream from Nita. Ellen and Tim hurried to their daughter. Then Tim saw the white stripe down the skunk's back as the animal turned and darted from the yard.

Ranger, their slick-haired dog, charged at the skunk and killed it. Tim got the animal away from the dog and put the thing in an empty room in the barn to dispose of later.

Ellen carried Nita into the house. After she had the kerosene lamp flickering, she saw that the animal had bitten her child on the chin and right arm. Blood appeared from both wounds. The distraught mother washed the wounds, then made a remedy of baking soda and kerosene and applied it to the broken skin. That was all she could do for the moment.

Ellen was awakened by a piercing scream from Nita. Then Tim saw the white stripe down the skunk's back as the animal turned and darted from the yard.

At daybreak Tim walked to the big house of the farmer for whom he was working that year. He woke a sleepy Henry Gibson and told him about the strange actions of the skunk which had bitten his child.

Henry seemed surprised. "Where did the skunk bite the girl?"

"On the chin and arm," Tim explained.

"Did the skunk discharge musk?"

"No. My dog killed the polecat after it had slipped onto the porch and attacked the child. The dog was in the back yard sleeping at the time."

"I'm afraid that skunk was rabid," Gibson said. "Such an animal will go for the victim's face. And rabid skunks rarely spray their foul scent. Must be hydrophobia."

Tim felt helpless. "What can we do for little Nita?"

"Doctors over at Commerce have a

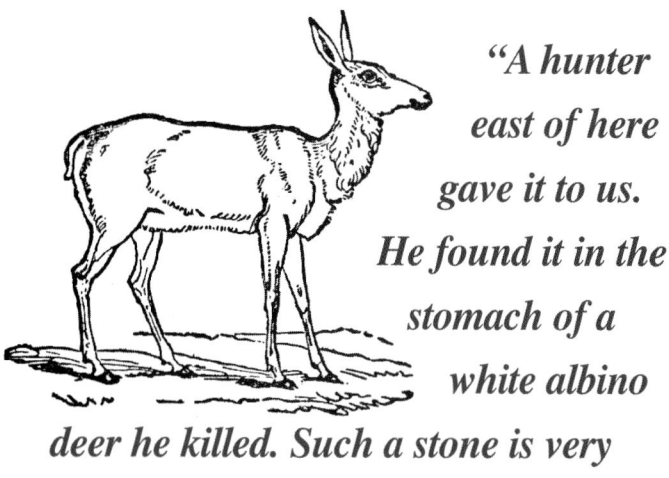

"A hunter east of here gave it to us. He found it in the stomach of a white albino deer he killed. Such a stone is very rare, as was that albino deer."

madstone, so I hear. You better rush the girl over to see those doctors. Name of Smith. Office's near the square."

Tim turned to leave. "Thanks. I'll get moving."

"Use my small buggy, Tim. Take care of little Nita."

A few minutes later Tim had his horse hitched to the buggy and his wife and child were ready for the long ride. They lived just west of Wolfe City in Hunt County. The doctors were 18 miles away.

Tim turned the buggy onto the main dirt highway and eased Charley into a fast trot. Nita crouched in her mother's arms, worried and afraid.

After they had traveled a mile, Ellen said, "We need to hurry." She seemed impatient with Tim and Charley.

"I know," Tim said. "But Charley has a long distance to travel. I don't want him to play out before we get to Commerce. We have to make it all the way. Charley will be exhausted when we finish the trip."

A few minutes later, Ellen realized Tim was right. The horse began to sweat in the hot, muggy weather. When they had traveled about 6 miles, Tim stopped and let Charley drink from a container he had brought for the horse. Charley then struck out in that fast trot, pulling the buggy easily.

Ellen sighed with relief and whispered a prayer three hours later when they entered Commerce. She felt sorry for Charley; the horse was covered with foamy sweat.

Tim found the doctors' office and carried Nita to see Dr. Wiley Smith. "I think our little girl was bitten by a rabid skunk. Can you help us?"

The doctor examined the wounds for a moment. Then he spoke comfortingly. "My brother Jimmy and I have a madstone. I can use it, and that is all the medical profession can do for you when a rabid animal has inflicted such a wound."

A few minutes later Nita was placed on a bed. The madstone was boiled in milk; then the doctor cooled it and placed it on the wound on Nita's arm. The stone seemed to stick there and the anxious parents prayed that the stone would draw the injection of the rabid skunk from their daughter.

The process of boiling the madstone and sticking it to the wounds was repeated throughout the afternoon and into the night. Then the stone fell free and would no longer stick to the wounds.

"That is all we can do," Dr. Smith explained. "The medical profession frowns on the use of a madstone, commonly called such because of mad dogs. Since we have no other remedy for rabies, we use the stone when someone thinks he has been bitten by a rabid animal."

"Where did you get the stone?" Tim asked.

"A hunter east of here gave it to us. He found it in the stomach of a white albino deer he killed. Such a stone is very rare, as was that albino deer."

"That is sort of a miracle," Tim said.

"Yes, especially if the porous stone has drawn all the rabies germs from your little daughter."

Tim picked up the stone and examined it. The rock had once been egg-shaped, but it had been cut so that the porous interior could be placed against a wound.

The next morning, Tim, Ellen and Nita got into the buggy. But this time Charley got to take his time.

Years passed. Nita always remembered the night that the skunk attacked her, the hurried trip to the doctor, and the work of the magical stone from the white deer.

Nita could never forget, for she always had a peculiar scar on her chin and right arm, mute evidence of the bites from the rabid skunk. ◆

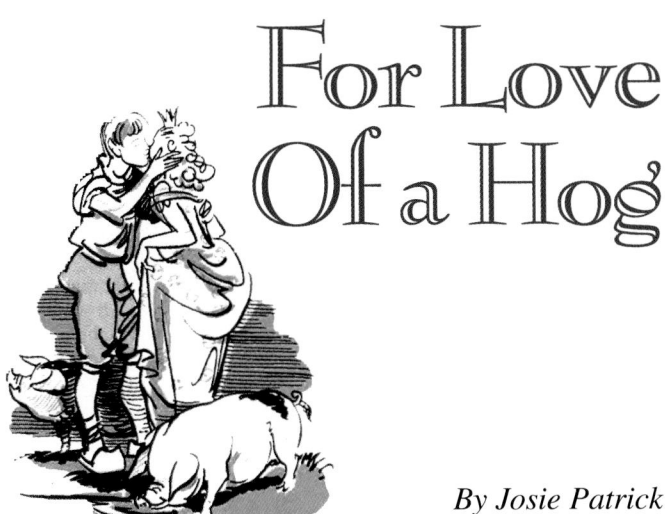

For Love Of a Hog

By Josie Patrick

Sister Pig was 5 years old and the pet of the family. My younger brother Tom, who came to love Sister Pig late, saw no fault in her after that day when she gobbled up the copperhead which was coiled, ready to strike him. Our hired hand, Lige, my brother Jim and I all adored her from the time she was the runt of the litter.

Whether snakes grew more plentiful or whether Sister Pig hunted them out, we never knew, but it became a not-infrequent sight to see Sister Pig chomping down on a snake. She'd jump upon it with her sharp hooves and break its body, along with its spirit. Then she'd start at its tail and eat it up almost before I could catch my breath.

"How does she do it, Jim?" I asked my older brother. He didn't know either.

The spring Sister Pig was 5, Lige got engaged to be married. Maude Jane was his girl's name, and though I was a little jealous, I had to admit she was pretty. She reminded me of a little pansy with her face peeping out from under a huge sunbonnet.

Maude Jane lived with her folks on the farm adjoining ours. Lige had lived with us for eight years, and he was just like part of the family—so much a part of it that I didn't see how we could ever do without him.

"You might as well get another ready," he said to her mother. "There sure is a lot of poison to draw out of there."

I worried that Lige would get married and leave us. Mama said he'd not leave at all. He'd just settle down on Mr. Ikey's place. (Mr. Ikey was Maude Jane's daddy.) To me, that wasn't the same at all. I couldn't see why Lige couldn't leave well enough alone—and that meant leaving Maude Jane alone. Mama said of course a 12-year-old girl like me couldn't expect to know how adults feel about such things, but that someday I would.

The wedding date was set for a Saturday night, Sept. 12. The wedding was going to be in our parlor. Mama helped Maude Jane make her wedding dress which was quite beautiful. It was as blue as the sky on a June day and the wide lace on it was as white as the sheets on Mama's clothesline on wash day.

For the occasion, Lige had a new suit, a new shirt and a new neck-tie. I watched him shine up his Sunday shoes and wondered how he could be as happy as the smile on his face said he was.

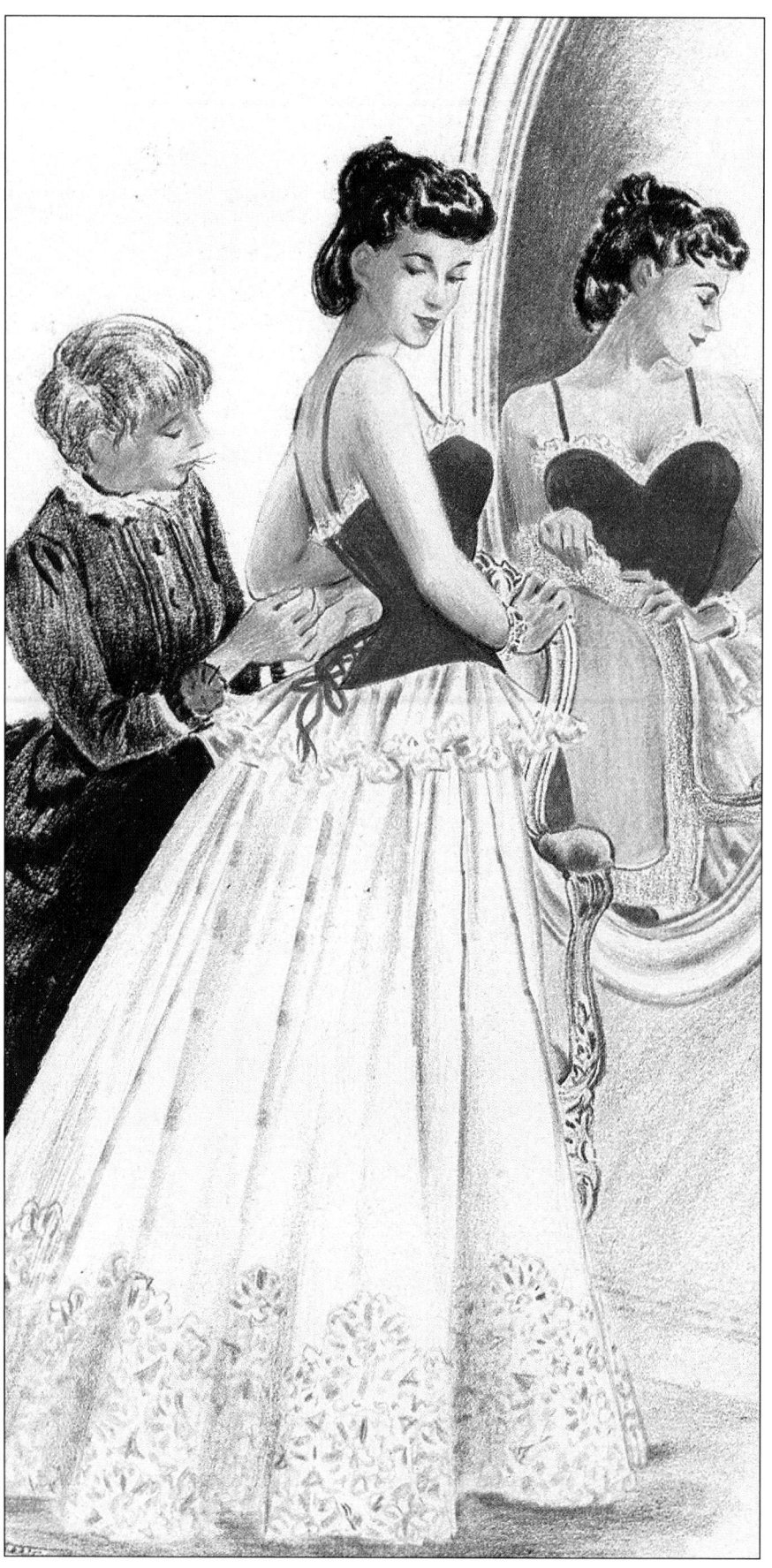

Late that afternoon Lige took a last look at Sister Pig. Then he went inside to get ready for his wedding. Sister Pig was going to have a litter and Lige was worried about her on account of her age.

When I went out a little later, I found Jim hovering over Sister Pig who was lying flat and grunting with every breath. "Run and get Lige," Jim begged. "Hurry. Sister Pig is bad off."

Maude Jane was already at our house, getting dressed in Mama's bedroom. Her folks would be coming over a little later. Brother Henson, who would perform the marriage, was in the kitchen drinking coffee with Papa.

I ran through the house calling for Lige. "Sister Pig's bad off. She needs you, Lige. Please come," I cried. Lige came, stuffing his shirt down into his breeches as he ran.

In a little while Maude Jane came out in her blue dress and high heels. "Lige," she cried, "if you think more of that old sow than you do of me, you can just marry her."

Lige didn't let on that he had heard her. He just went on helping Sister Pig. Maude Jane turned and stomped away, her high heels fairly flying over the ground.

Three hours later Sister Pig had eight little piglets. They were as squirmy and healthy as they could be. Sister Pig lay resting, a satisfied grin on her face.

Lige realized now that he should have been married by this time. He jumped up and ran toward the house, his shirttail flying like a kite.

Mama was in the parlor. So were Papa and the preacher. But Maude Jane had gone home.

"She was awfully angry, Lige," Brother Henson said. "She said since you'd left your wedding to go to Sister Pig, she guessed there would be no wedding."

"Well, if she's going to be like that ..." Lige was busy stuffing his shirttail inside his breeches.

We were all just sitting there, feeling sad—even me, when I saw how crestfallen Lige was—when a loud knock came at the door. Mr. Ikey burst in.

"Can one of you go for the doctor for me quick?" he asked. "Maude Jane stepped on a snake on her way home and it bit her. Her ankle looks like a log, it's swollen so big." He glared at Lige. "And it's all your fault. If you'd been in here attending to your business, it never would have happened."

Papa jumped up. "I'll go for the doctor," he said.

"And I'll go with you," Brother Henson told Mr. Ikey. "Maude Jane and her mother may need us."

"I'll go along too," Lige said. "But I doubt that Maude Jane will see me."

I tagged along. I was feeling so bad about Maude Jane being mad at Lige. I was trying to think of something to say to her.

Maude Jane was lying on the couch, groaning. Her ankle was twice the normal size.

"Gosh!" Lige said. "We can't wait for that doctor. He's 10 miles away. He won't be here for an hour and a half at least." He knelt beside Maude Jane, then turned to Mrs. Ikey. "Go and get one of your fryers," he told her.

In a few minutes Mrs. Ikey was back with the chicken; she'd already wrung its neck. Lige took a knife and split it down the middle. He pulled out the insides, then wrapped the still-warm fowl around Maude Jane's ankle. "You might as well get another ready," he said to her mother. "There sure is a lot of poison to draw out of there."

In half an hour Lige removed the first chicken. Its flesh was tinged with green. "Look at that poison," Mrs. Ikey said. "How do you

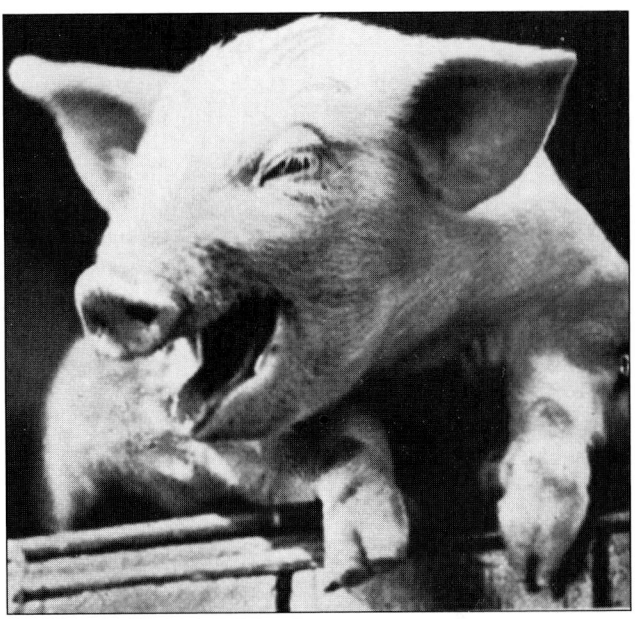

feel, daughter?"

"Better. It doesn't pain so much," Maude Jane replied.

"Hand me the other chicken." Lige wrapped it lovingly around her ankle. "Burn this one." He handed Mrs. Ikey the first chicken. "All that old snake's poison went into it."

"Oh, Lige, you know everything." Maude Jane looked up at him and smiled.

"I'm sorry about this evening, Maude Jane," Lige said. "I hope you'll forgive me. But Sister Pig was in trouble. I just had to help her."

"Oh, I guess I was just jealous," Maude Jane laughed. "I know she needed you. And that's the kind of person you are, Lige. I guess ..." She blushed. "I guess that's why I love you. You can be depended on."

Lige kissed her on the forehead. "Guess what? Sister Pig has eight little piglets."

"Like her?" Maude Jane asked.

"Well, I hope so," he replied. "If they eat snakes like their mama does, these parts will be well rid of them."

Papa burst through the doorway. "The doctor's gone into the next county to deliver a baby. We can't get ahold of him till morning."

"We don't need him," Mr. Ikey said.

"Lige has taken care of everything," Brother Henson said.

"You bet." Maude kept looking at Lige and smiling. ◆

Warts

By Edgar Harrison

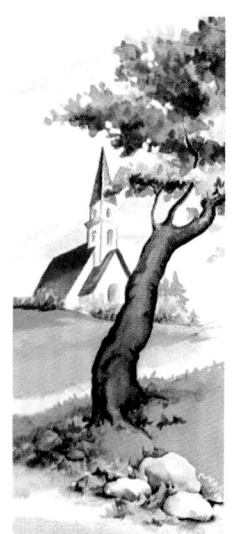

I suppose most folks have had a wart at some time. Those pesky bumps annoy a person until he takes action to get rid of them.

In our community, there was an old fellow who claimed to be a wizard. Supposedly he could work a number of everyday miracles, such as charming off warts.

One Sunday after church, I approached him with a wart I had on the knuckle of my right index finger. It was ugly and bled a lot. I'd tried taking it off with everything from shoe polish to horse liniment, but it stubbornly remained. The wart wizard was my last hope.

He squinted at my proffered finger. "You've been pickin' at that," he observed. "You'd better stop that or it'll spread. You came to me just in time.

"I've got two methods of takin' off warts. The most foolproof requires that you wash the wart with spunk water out of a stump at midnight, saying incantations." He looked at me closely. "Your mama let you out of the house after dark like that?"

Reluctantly, I allowed as how that was not likely.

"Well, alright," he said. "The other method works, too. I guess I'll just have to buy your wart. I'll have what I need next Sunday. You be here."

Needless to say, during the next week I was consumed by curiosity. I questioned every boy I knew. Some admitted to having had their warts removed by the wart wizard, but they all remained suspiciously silent about the process.

By the following Sunday, my anxiety level had reached epidemic proportions. I worried through the church service and I even contemplated sneaking away afterward without seeing him, but he was waiting at the back of the church.

"Meet me beside the men's outhouse," he whispered, "and don't let anyone see you!" Then he lined up to shake hands with the preacher.

I looked around furtively. Since no one was paying much attention to me, I slipped out the side door and ran around behind the building. With the pungent odor of the outhouse wafting around me, I nervously waited for the wizard.

With many sidelong glances, he slunk alongside of me, grabbed my shoulder and pulled me behind the outhouse.

"Where's your wart?" he demanded. I stuck out my finger. From his pants pocket, he produced a shiny new penny. He rubbed it over the wart, reciting solemnly:

"Come to me, wart,
"You are mine!
"I purchased you
"For a dollar ninety-nine!"

He handed the penny to me. "I've bought your wart," he said. "In a few days, it'll drop off and come to me."

"But you said in the poem, 'a dollar ninety-nine'! Will the wart come off for a penny?" I asked.

"Warts can't count," he said, and winked at me. Then he grabbed my arm again. "If you ever tell a soul what went on back here, this is what'll happen to you!" He pulled down his shirt collar to reveal a hairy shoulder almost entirely covered with warts. I quickly crossed my heart.

He was right. In a few days my wart fell off. Whether the wart wizard grew another bump on his back, I'll never know.

That wart never returned until about a year ago. At that time I asked our newly graduated young doctor for a cure.

"There's only one cure I know of that really works," he told me. "You take a potato and cut it in half. Rub both sides on the wart and bury it at midnight while reciting...." ◆

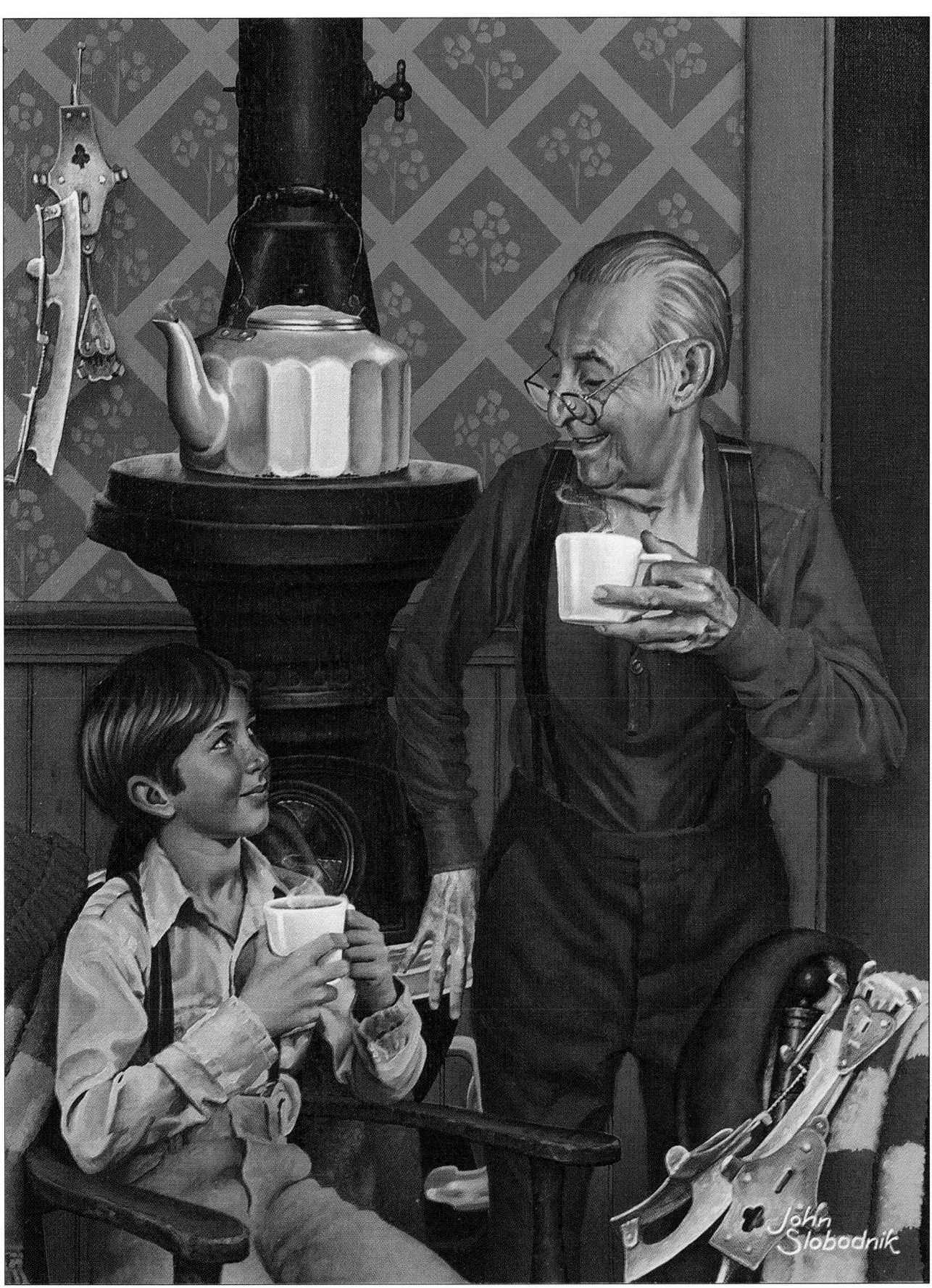

Grandma's Secret

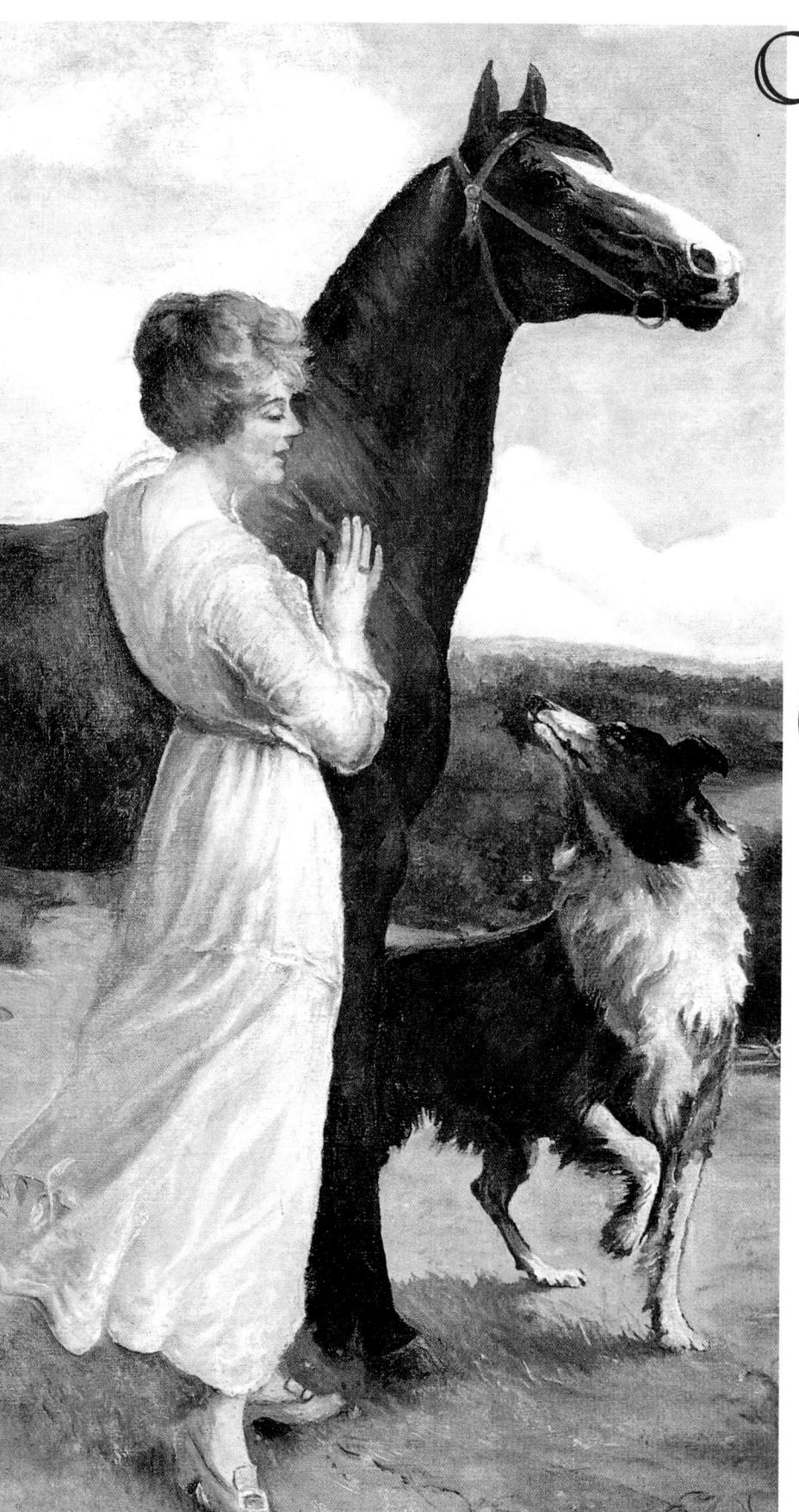

By Yulene A. Rushton

Grandma wouldn't tell me and boy, was I mad! I wanted to know, and I was determined to find out. I had propped myself on top of the wooden claw feet under the kitchen table, concealed by the red-and-white checkered oilcloth which hung halfway to the floor. I listened intently, scarcely breathing, afraid I'd miss what I was hoping to hear.

His faded pantlegs and scuffed leather boots were visible, but I couldn't see anything more of Ellis Holman. I knew he was sitting sprawl-legged on a chair watching Grandma. Her black lace-up shoes clicked across the linoleum floor from where she had silently stood at the cupboard, doing something with a small piece of cloth.

I heard her say, "Now Ellis, I don't want you to think about your wart ever again. If you think about it, it won't go away. Sometime after you've forgotten completely, you'll look and it will be gone." I knew Ellis must be nodding in agreement because he didn't utter a word.

Darn! I thought. *She told him the same thing she told me, and he's more grown-up. I thought she'd tell something extra.*

I crouched in my hiding place, envisioning Grandma as some sort of kind witch with magical powers. I could hardly stand not knowing, but I was not to learn the secret yet.

Repeated coaxing would not make Grandma reveal the formula she had been given by her grandmother years before. I persisted in my pleading until one day she finally promised, "Yulene my dear, when I am ready to give up my power to charm away warts, I can tell only one person. When that time comes, you will be the one whom I will tell. Leave it be, now! Quit pestering me, or you'll never know!" There was a twinkle in her eye but a firmness in her voice. I knew she meant it, and I conceded to being satisfied with eager anticipation, awaiting the time when I would know what only she could tell.

Over the years I watched with great interest every time an occasional person came to her door. The door would close and shortly the two of them would come out smiling and silent. I knew what they were up to and I felt important with the knowledge that someday I'd be the charmer.

I grew older and married. I temporarily forgot about the secret. Then, while I was visiting Grandma one day, she motioned me into the kitchen. The door clicked shut behind us. "I'm getting old and tired," Grandma said. "I'm going to tell you a secret today." As she smiled, *Warts!* flashed into my mind.

Excitement surged through me and I listened very carefully. But I thought I had missed something. Grandma repeated the instructions a second time. I remember thinking, *Can it be that simple?*

"Are you sure that's all there is to it?" I asked her. "Don't you mix some rare, complicated, magical witch's potion or something?"

Grandma chuckled. "It's worked for me all

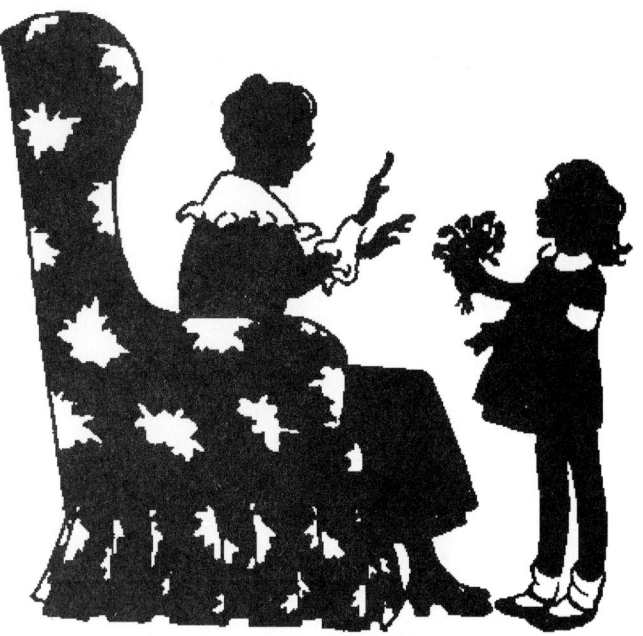

I could hardly stand not knowing, but I was not to learn the secret yet.

these years, and it will for you, too. But never, never tell a soul until you're ready to pass along the secret to just one other person." She hugged me and mumbled something about her firstborn sweetheart of a granddaughter.

I left her home feeling a bit disappointed in what she had told me, but filled with excitement about my new role as "wart charmer." I told everyone about Grandma giving her secret to me, and anxiously waited for someone to get a wart they would be willing to part with.

Nervously I wondering if this was considered witchcraft. I didn't want to be run out of town or, even worse, burned at the stake. I talked myself into thinking that there was nothing wrong with it. After all, I wasn't an old hag who flew through the October sky on a broomstick, and I wasn't doing evil or anything of a harmful nature. I was simply trying to help people rid themselves of an obnoxious presence in their lives. I reasoned that if I *was* tinkering on the edge of witchery, then I must be one of those good, kind witches.

It seemed forever until that day when my

young nephew Brad came by, proudly sporting a big bump on his thumb. "I got this from Timmy, a big toad I caught in the field," he said. "Mama says it's ugly and I should tell you to wish it away." The expression on his freckled face told me that he wasn't so sure he wanted to get rid of it. But that same expression was also challenging my newfound powers. He was anxious to know if Auntie was really a "wart wisher-offer."

As I had seen Grandma do so many times, I took him into my kitchen, closed the door, and proceeded to follow her instructions. I heard my voice speaking in low, reassuring tones. "Don't think about this wart, ignore it, and don't mention it to a living soul. One day you'll look and it will be gone. You have to believe!" Then I sent him on his way. We were both anxious, wondering if this mysterious nonsense would work.

It did. And over the next few years, many more visited my kitchen. I never stopped being amazed at this strange phenomenon.

At times I was a little embarrassed to be referred to as "the lady I told you about who wishes away warts." Somehow I wanted to be known for something a little more special than a thing like that.

Del Ashby, a gray-haired and good-natured co-worker, had a wart on his finger just where his pencil fit. He worked as a bookkeeper so it was an awful nuisance to him. He had tried all sorts of remedies from the pharmacy, but to no avail. He laughed when I told him, "I can get rid of that thing for you." But finally, in desperation, one day he asked me to try my secret charms on him. I obliged, and a few weeks later I commented, "Del, I notice your wart is gone."

"Yeah," he replied, "but it was probably some of the stuff I daubed on it before I came to see you."

I made no comment, but smiled. *Let him believe what he will,* I thought.

Occasionally the secret method didn't work, but I was convinced then that the warted person had a big mouth and hadn't kept quiet like he was supposed to. That was a big part of the remedy.

Probably the most outstanding experience I ever had with the lumpy menaces was an episode with our horse, Koko. I don't know how often a horse comes down with warts, but at one time Koko sported at least a hundred. They covered his nose, mouth and parts of his face. His soft, velvety nose was bumpy and ugly, and it felt strange to the touch as he nuzzled for grain and sugar lumps.

We tried salves and medicines recommended by our veterinarian, but to our dismay, none of them worked. Jokingly, my husband, Norm, commented, "The only thing we haven't tried is wishing them off. How about it?"

"Are you kidding?" I responded. "Wish warts off a horse?"

"Why not? It works on people. And I'm sure he won't tell!"

"Well, why not?" I shrugged. I gathered the things I needed and tramped out to the corral to perform my magic on Koko. I whispered in his ear as if he were a person while I performed the little ritual of Grandma's secret.

It was hard not to think about Koko's apparent ailment because his nose twitched back and forth in such a noticeable fashion whenever he chewed his daily portion of hay. We tried not to watch, and waited.

One day Norm came in with a puzzled look on his face. "Can you beat that?" he said. " Koko's warts are gone!" With raised eyebrows and wide eyes, my amazement was difficult to hide.

It has been years now since I have used my power to charm warts. People don't seem to get warts nearly as often as they used to. In fact, hardly anyone I know has had one for a long, long time.

Now I am the grandma who will probably pass the secret on to a curious grandchild who may be silently wondering if I am a kind witch who delves into unexplainable magic.

As I reflect on this strange power, I'm convinced that it is a power of the mind, metaphysical, probably linked to the power of suggestion and positive thinking. Nevertheless, it works, and the secret has come full circle.... ◆

First Aid at Home

By Herschel L. Smith

On the farm, our medicine cabinet was well-stocked for humans and animals. We had red liniment for humans and black liniment for animals. The black liniment was mighty strong—too strong to rub on human skin. Both liniments were good for treating sprains, lacerations and bruises.

There was also a bottle of peroxide. The peroxide foamed when it was applied to open wounds, and this made it appear to be death on germs.

Besides different patent medicines we had home emergency treatments peculiar to our community. The local cure for a snakebite was to kill a black chicken, cut it open and apply some of the still-warm innards to the wound immediately.

We knew about tourniquets to stop bleeding, but we also had something—or *someone*—special. An old man who lived about a mile from us had inherited the mysterious ability to stop bleeding in animals and humans by some spiritual means. He used the Bible. Some of our neighbors swore by this, but I don't recall that we ever used his services.

The home remedy which impressed me most was used to treat puncture wounds to insure that they wouldn't become infected. A cylinder of a waxy substance about 3 inches long and ¾ inch in diameter was held over a coal-oil lamp to melt. The hot wax was smeared on a clean white cloth, and while the wax was still quite warm, the cloth was pasted over the puncture wound. The next morning, we could be sure that the wax over the wound would be green.

We frequently used this treatment on puncture wounds caused by rusty nails, and infection never developed. But I don't remember the name of the waxy substance.

At least once or twice a year, Dad would get supplies for his medicine cabinet from a huckster who drove an enclosed horse-drawn wagon. For us, that wagon was a drugstore on wheels! In those days, going to the hospital was absolutely the last resort, as was seeing the family doctor. ◆

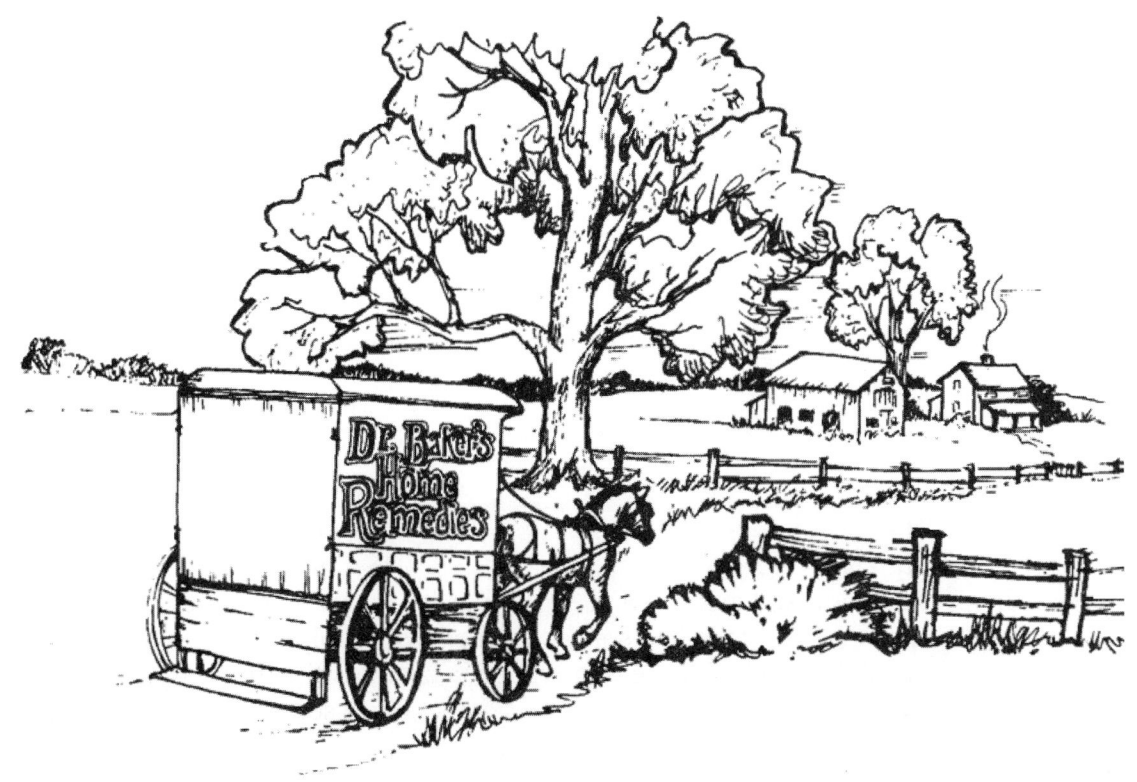

Ozark Medicine

By J. Whittemore

I often think of the days when I was growing up in the beautiful Arkansas Ozarks. How lucky I was to have lived at a time when a garden-fresh tomato tasted like the good Lord intended it to taste, when apples were not glazed with wax, and when water from a well could quench one's thirst like no other beverage devised by man.

I also think of the lady who possibly saved my life when I was a child. She was known as Aunt Sadie, although she was nobody's aunt in particular. I have no idea how many births, weddings and deaths came and went under her jurisdiction, but there were a great many. She was an expert nurse and practiced medicine freely without formal education or a license.

In her spare time, she collected all sorts of amazingly useful roots and herbs. Doc Slocum, the regular country doctor, never objected when Aunt Sadie was called in. He probably realized that her natural gift for nursing would help.

In 1921, our community was besieged by a terrible epidemic of scarlet fever, and I caught it. There were no antibiotics in those days, and in an epidemic, the organism which caused it just grew stronger and stronger. Many country children died.

One day I complained to my mother of a sore throat and headache, and I began to run a fever. Dad called in the family doctor, and when he peered into my mouth and observed my "strawberry tongue," he shook his head sadly.

"Is it scarlet?" my mother asked.

"I'm afraid so," Doc Slocum replied. He opened his black bag and gave me some sort of pill. My mother bathed me with alcohol but my fever raged on. Dad, who was a vet, knew all about four-legged animals but nothing about human diseases. Both Mom and Dad were very worried. I was their only child—and probably a very spoiled one.

Finally, Mom hesitatingly asked Doc Slocum if he would be offended if they called in Aunt Sadie.

How lucky I was to have lived at a time when a garden-fresh tomato tasted like the good Lord intended it to taste!

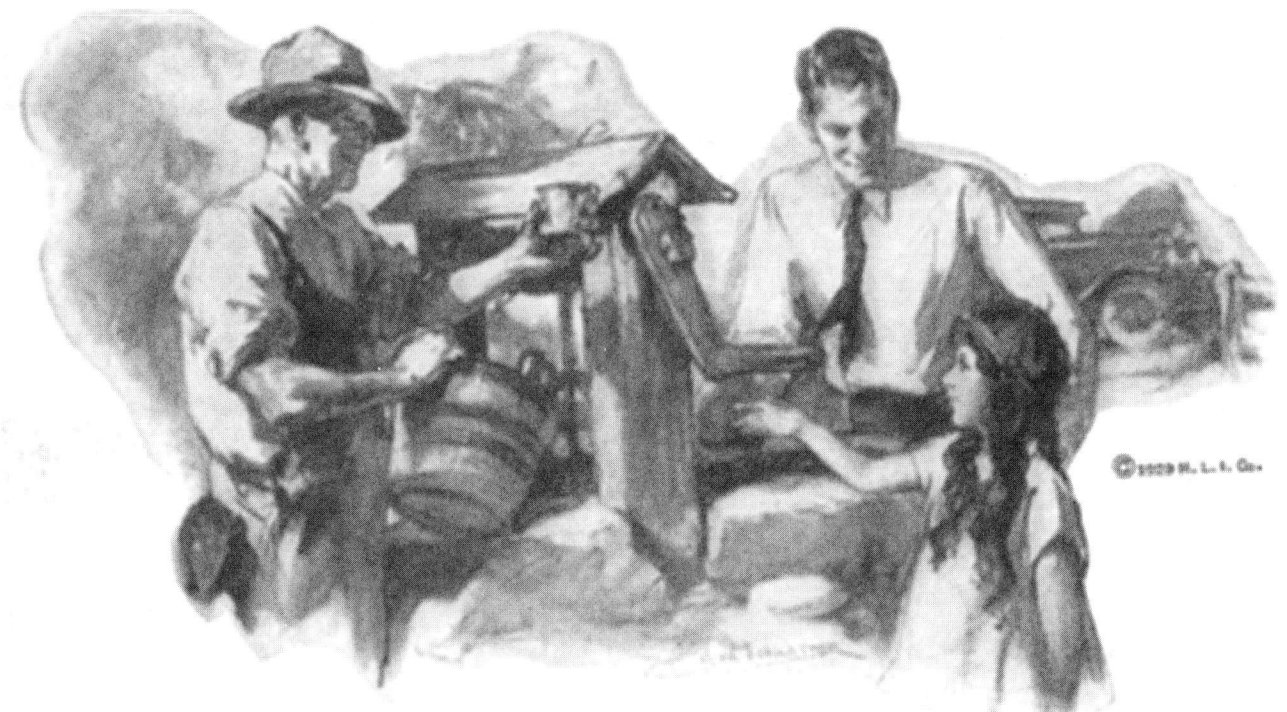

When I was growing up in the Arkansas Ozarks, water from a well could quench one's thirst like no other beverage devised by man.

"Go right ahead," replied old Doc. "She can't do any harm, and if she has some trick in that parcel of herbs she carries around that will help, I'm all for it."

So as not to waste time, Dad drove over to Aunt Sadie's in the Model T, and returned a short time later with the local "yarb gatherer." She felt my chest with her motherly hand and made me partake of one of her mysterious brews.

"Jest to be on the safe side," she remarked to my mother, "I think we should change her name. That way, the angel of death will think he's got the wrong customer."

"Anything you say," my mother replied. She was so distracted by worry that she would have agreed to anything.

"In that case," Aunt Sadie said, "her name is no longer Jessie."

Then she dropped to her knees beside my bed. "Dear Lord," she began, "I would like to baptize this dear little girl whose name is Mary Ann Whittemore." Sprinkling some water on my fevered brow, she continued: "In the name of the Father, Son and Holy Ghost, I baptize

this dear little girl, Mary Ann Whittemore. Please, dear Lord, help her to grow up a Christian who will always love her neighbor and do her best to follow in the path of Your Son, Jesus. Thank you, Lord. Amen."

Aunt Sadie got to her feet and said to my mother, "This here new daughter you've got, Mary Ann Whittemore, is a fine girl. One of these days maybe I'll be on hand when she gets married."

In a few hours my temperature began to return to normal. With good nursing care from Aunt Sadie and my mother, I made a complete recovery.

Later on, Doc Slocum told my dad that Aunt Sadie exerted a strange effect on a child's mind which seemed to help. Perhaps I would have recovered anyway, but the people in our community believed that Aunt Sadie possessed a certain magic.

A few days after my "baptism," I asked my mother when I could go back to my old name.

"I don't know, child," she replied. "We'll have to ask Aunt Sadie." ◆

Aunt Hattie's Love Rash

By Carl Wolfgang Maiwald

The mysterious ailment started when my Aunt Hattie was 27. It was all Ira Pellou's fault—or so it would seem. And, there could be only one miracle cure for what ailed her.

Aunt Hattie was my mother's oldest sister and lived at home with my grandparents. Ira was a happy, hulking woodchopper who worked for the Kalter and Bettelmann Lumber Company. His courting of Hattie consisted of "dropping in" at Grandpa's farm every Sunday, just about when the dinner bell rang.

After a gargantuan meal—besides pies, salads and such trifles, he'd put away a whole chicken plus a huge mound of mashed Irish potatoes doused in gravy—Ira would take Hattie to a picnic or a church sociable in his "trusty" Model T. Afterward, he'd usually take her to the Show Shop, a livery stable which had been converted into a movie house.

On their very first date Hattie had a slight itch in her left palm. It vanished overnight, so she forgot it—until it came back, stronger, on the second date. On their third date, the itch was so bad that Ira noticed Hattie digging at her hand, and asked her why. "Oh, it's nothing probably. What does it mean when your left hand itches? Oh look, the Keystone Cops are stalled on the railroad tracks," Hattie replied to divert his attention.

But Ira had a one-track mind. "Money. It means money, folks say."

Hattie disagreed. "Papa says, 'Kiss a fool; meet a stranger; or some poor devil's neck is in danger.' Hey! Stop it! What's got into you?"

"Well, you said 'Kiss a fool.' I don't mind being that fool."

Hattie blushed to the roots of her hair. "Shush. People are staring. Keep your mind on the show."

When Ira had *putt-putted* away in his Lizzie for another dreadfully long week, Hattie rubbed cold cream into her hand. By morning the itch was gone, but on her next date it came on stronger and lasted longer.

As the romance progressed, so did the malady. All manner of salves and lotions were tried, but only the one her Pa suggested helped. It was a thick grease called Bag Balm and was mainly for cows, but he claimed it to be "good for man or beast."

The red, sore, itching rash would go away during the week. But come Sunday and come Ira, it would strike again. Dr. Metcalf was consulted, but the ointments he prescribed did no good; in fact, it spread to her other hand, too.

Finally the doctor, Grandma, Hattie and my mother became convinced that Hattie was allergic to Ira. When they told Ira of their diagnosis, he admitted he might be the cause of the pernicious ailment, but felt it was intense love and not an allergy that caused the trouble. Still, he nobly volunteered to give up the gal. The womenfolk shed many tears. Even Ira—all 250 brawny pounds of him—had to keep blowing his nose, using his red bandanna as a cover-up.

Grandpa took no part in the waterworks. He was a smart old codger and realized that at 27, Hattie had an excellent chance of becoming an old maid. Thinking of all the time and big dinners invested in Ira, he spoke up.

"Why don't you young folks just up and get hitched? Soon as you are together every blessed day, the itch will go away. I guarantee it! As I see it, Ira is man enough to end the misery he's causing my daughter. And I couldn't ask for a better son-in-law. Right, Ira?"

Well, there was a hasty wedding, though not for the reason some nosy gossips hinted, for they were married for a year and a half before Ira, Jr., made his appearance. Theirs was a good marriage, and it produced six cousins of mine.

It wasn't until Uncle Ira's funeral last year that I mentioned Aunt Hattie's "love rash" to her.

Her smile lit up her musty parlor as we sat side by side on the horsehair sofa. She patted the nude spot on my head the way she used to pat the thick mop which once grew there. "Love, my eye," she said, giving me a conspiratorial wink.

"That's what it was, Aunt Hattie. Mother has told me that story many times."

"Not the whole story, darling boy." (I was 50 at the time.) "I promised your grandpa we'd keep our little secret as long as Ira was alive, but it wasn't love that made that pesky rash. It was potatoes."

"Potatoes?" I parroted the word without understanding.

The red, sore, itching rash would go away during the week. But come Sunday and come Ira, it would strike again.

"Yes, Carl. Potatoes, spuds, tubers. You see, during the week we cooked them in their skins, but when Ira called, my mother would fix his favorite mashed potatoes. I'd peel a heap of them every Sunday morning. The juice would soak into my hands, and by the time we got to the movies, I'd start to break out."

"But how did you find out and how did marrying Uncle Ira cure you?"

"Your grandpa figured it out."

"Didn't he tell you?" I asked indignantly.

"Yes, but he asked me to bear up until I got married. He didn't want any slip-up."

"Well, every time I had dinner at your table, we had mashed potatoes," I remembered. "So you never stopped peeling potatoes."

"Of course not. Ira didn't care for spuds boiled in their jackets, but there's more than one way to skin a potato. Your grandpa had a bright idea."

"Such as," I hinted.

She gave me a sly grin. "Along with the 10 cows my pa gave us to set up farming, he gave me a little wedding present."

"An electric potato peeler?" I asked.

"A 25-cent pair of rubber gloves," she smiled. ◆

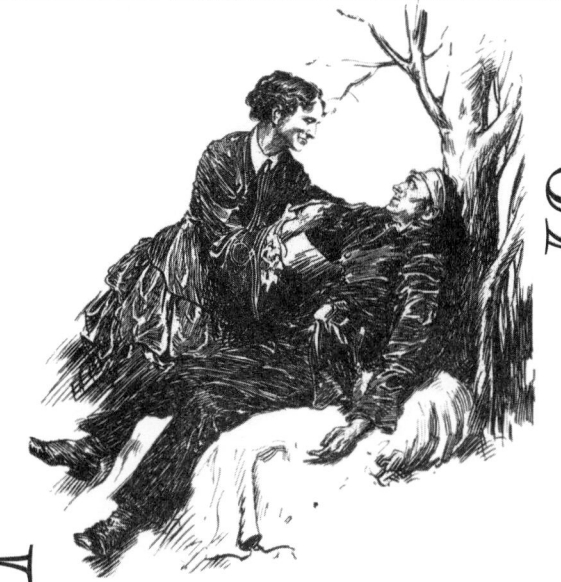

Blood Stoppers

ditor's Note: "First Aid at Home" refers to an old man who could stop bleeding. In the old days, when doctors were as rare as hen's teeth in rural and frontier areas, many regions had such people who were, whether by fact or lore, endowed with the ability to stop bleeding by word, touch or other action. They were commonly known as "blood stoppers." Back in 1995 I asked readers of *Good Old Days* magazine to send me their memories of blood stoppers; we received an avalanche of mail from all over North America, all attesting to the veracity of the blood stopper tales. Few books have documented this lore; here are some of their stories:

In the old days, when doctors were rare, many regions had people who were, whether by fact or lore, endowed with the ability to stop bleeding.

When I was a child we had a man in our neighborhood named Henry. He could stop bleeding.

He memorized and said or read Ezekiel 16:6 from the Bible: "And when I passed by thee, and saw thee polluted in thine own blood, I said unto thee when thou wast in thy blood, Live; yea, I said unto thee when thou wast in thy blood, Live."

I don't know if he had a prayer with that or not.

Our Bible was marked: "To stop blood read Ezekiel 16:6." We never had an occasion to use the cure.

Mrs. Harvey Baker, Fredericktown, Mo.

I have heard of blood stoppers, and was healed once by one. I was born and reared at Friday, Texas, and remember once when a farm animal was cut badly with barbed wire.

A lady in the community was contacted. I know she was never around the animal, but the bleeding stopped.

Now it might have ceased anyway; I simply don't know. I wouldn't try to analyze it.

As I remember, this was a carefully kept secret, held by the person who could stop bleeding.

Velma Warner, Galena Park, Texas

My father was a blood stopper. We lived on a creek in eastern Kentucky. If someone got hurt in the mines or while logging, they sent word to my father as soon as they could.

I remember people saying they knew the minute Dad got word, the blood would stop—like you had just turned it off.

When I was in my 20s, Dad told me how to do it. There were four of us girls, so I don't know why he picked me.

I never had to try it, and had just forgotten about it until I read the letter in *Good Old Days*.

Bonnie Caldwell, Morrow, Ohio

My mother could stop blood. She would say a verse from the Bible as she held the wound.

A blood stopper cannot pass the information on to their spouse, a blood relative, or a member of the same sex. Otherwise they themselves would lose the power.

I know it works, as I have seen my mother do it a number of times. She died last spring at the age of 80. She told my husband the verse and how to stop blood before she died.

Mrs. M.J. Robinson, Pikeville, Ky.

Blood stoppers use the Bible and also cobwebs that form in everyone's home. We always kept one large cobweb for that purpose.

I have written instructions for stopping bleeding passed down from over 150 years ago. Like all our gifts it goes from woman to man to woman, and if it's not done this way you lose the gift.

The cobweb is applied directly to the source of the bleeding and Ezekiel 16:6 is recited.

We blow out fire from burns and cure short growth with words handed down through the ages in our family. I'm half Irish and half Cherokee and I use and believe in a lot of old-time medicines.

Helen Watts, Mattoon, Ill.

You don't have to believe it if you don't want to, but an old Canadian Indian told me: "Go in the barn, and upon the high rafters and get a gob of cobwebs and lay them on the wound."

I turned 81 in March. When I was 4 I cut the bottom of my foot badly on a piece of glass. My dad pulled it out and tied a piece of salt pork on. In a few days he took it off. The wound was all healed.

Edward Rumrill, Springfield, Vt.

In Rhode Island, as I grew up in the late '20s and early '30s there were several blood stoppers.

The French-Canadian immigrants thought that the men who were the seventh sons of a seventh son had the power to control profuse bleeding, among other things.

Twice during this period I experienced injuries where I bled profusely. Both times one of my dad's employees was brought to stop the bleeding.

I will always remember this elderly gentleman because of how gentle and humble he was. He spoke softly and touched the bleeding area while asking if I felt an "aura" of heat, which I did both times.

The bleeding stopped almost immediately.

The man was often called upon by the local doctors to assist them in cases where there were injuries resulting in profuse bleeding.

He would never accept money or other recompense from those whom he helped.

Dr. Gil Mongeau, West Warwick, R.I.

Although I have no firsthand experience with this, my maternal grandmother possessed this ability. She died in 1929.

The one thing I recall was there could't be water between the flow of blood and Grandmother.

Unfortunately, my mother has been gone since 1988. I do recall Mother saying that Grandmother could only pass the gift to her oldest child, but never got it done.

Phil Frisbie, Vestaburg, Mich.

I lived in the Great Smoky Mountains in my young days. We didn't have doctors or hospitals; we depended on herbs and home remedies, like the blood stoppers.

My mother cut her foot badly, and I was sent to my aunt's house to get her to stop the bleeding.

I wanted her to come back with me because I thought she had to see the cut first. She said for me to run back to my mother. When I got home the bleeding had already stopped. My aunt used a verse from Ezekiel. Anyone can stop bleeding if they have the faith it will work.

Edna Welch, Marion, N.C.

Old-Time Remedies

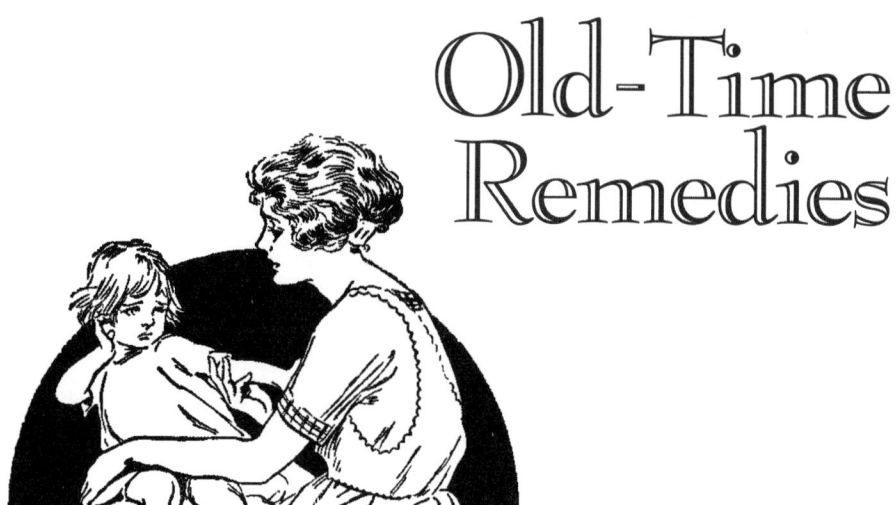

I remember dad with his "dental kit"—a piece of string, a diverting story, and a doorknob. The string was tied to the tooth and then to the knob and a story was told to you. The synopsis of the story was "You won't feel a thing," and surprisingly enough, I didn't. My confidence in Dad was reestablished, and sometime during the night I was visited by a benevolent new friend, the tooth fairy.

My grandmother had a great home remedy for removing warts. You were directed to take a potato and to put a penny into it for each wart you had; then, believe it or not, you were to hide it and forget where you hid it.

Edward W. Thomas

My mother used to give it to us kids, and even though we didn't like to take it, she made us.

I was born with asthma, and when we moved to the Canadian Maritimes, my condition was made much worse by the dampness. The rural doctors could not give strong enough medication to control my asthma.

I was close to dying one night when the local witch doctor showed up at the door. You never had to call this lady—she just showed up when needed.

She immediately asked for some old newspapers and made me a paper jacket "to draw off the dampness from the chest." I felt better immediately. The jackets were changed as soon as they felt damp. I still place a newspaper over my chest for asthma attacks, and it still works.

Alan Whidden, Babb, Mont.

For children with lung trouble like asthma, cut a sourwood stick the length of the child and put it in the closet or anywhere near where the child lives. Sourwood flowers are what bees make honey from. We have a lot of it in South Carolina. It will work for as long as a person is growing. That's all there is to it—no hoax or sham.

Mable Chasteen, Greenville, S.C.

I was raised in a family of nine children. I am the only one left of them, being the youngest. I am 84 and in very good health. For diarrhea and stomach pain, take 1 heaping tablespoon of white flour in a small drinking glass of water. Mix well and drink fast. It will cure diarrhea and stomach pain in less than two minutes. If the ache persists, repeat the dosage. It never fails.

My mother used to give it to us kids, and even though we didn't like to take it, she made us.

John Hinds, Lynnwood, Wash

To remedy snake bite, first of all find some means of very greatly arousing the activities of the various purifying organs of the body. Probably the first method would be to drink large quantities of hot water, as much as your stomach will hold. If hot water is not available, cold water is better than nothing. A steam bath would be especially valuable; also a hot wet sheet pack, inducing profuse perspiration. The lower bowel should also be cleansed by the injection of as much hot water as one can retain. Of course, all of this treatment should not necessarily be given at the same time, for it might in itself cause death, but as much as a patient can stand.

—From 1910

Poor eyesight is often due to improper mastication to the extent that a fault of this kind would lessen general vitality. The strength of one's eyes depends largely on the strength of the body throughout; in other words, if you are strong muscularly and vitally, your eyes will be strong. Eyes are nourished by the blood the same as any other tissues of the body, and an improved quality of blood means improved eyesight. Those afflictions that are ordinarily supposed to require glasses can be remedied in practically every instance by adding to the vitality of the general system, and giving the eyes the benefit of certain methods such as eye baths and eye exercises.

—From 1910

Friction applied by the hands will help a numb condition in the legs. Also, rubbing with a coarse brush or towel will improve circulation and relieve the numb sensation. It is caused by imperfect circulation and impaired nutrition for nerves. It may arise from defective digestion and excess of acid in the blood.

—From 1913

Chronic disease like asthma will not let go easily. It cannot be poisoned out with drugging. What is drugging but poisoning? Every drug is a poison, even soda or magnesia. Some drugs will deaden sensation and mislead a person into thinking he is relieved. Actually, asthma is a result of imperfect digestion. It will be well to eat rice, bread and fruit, apples and oranges, potato and asparagus, and drink only water. Also, the body will suffer less if the skin is always warm and dry.

—From 1913

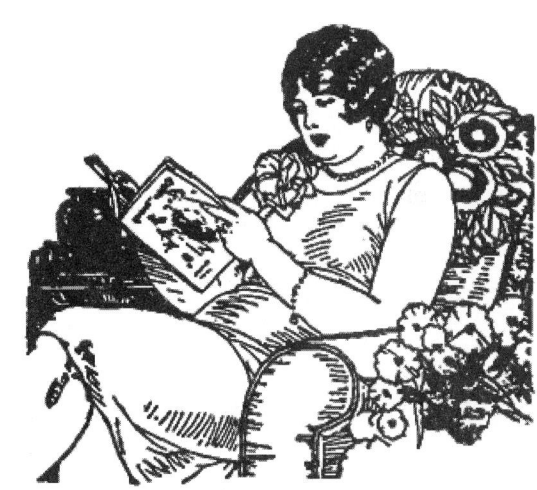

Why The Posture of the Body Is Important

1. Form is the concrete, tangible expression of an idea.

2. Correct posture is the physical manifestation of culture and breeding.

3. Form, though a reflex product, reacts upon the wearer.

4. Form acts as the rail upon a car-wheel; it guides properly or improperly according to the form.

5. Society protects itself by demanding the observance of a standard of good form.

6. A contracted body spells fear and suspicion. A flabby body spells self-indulgence and laziness. Expanded and erect muscles spell love and faith, both in ourselves and in our fellow-men.

7. Correct posture is a conservator of energy, and assures the maximum of efficiency with the minimum of effort.

—From 1910

Those Old-Time Cures

By Ruth Florea Collins

People my age can thank their lucky stars that they not only survived the childhood illnesses which all children seem to get, but also survived the remedies which were often applied to cure them.

At our house, only a few regular medicines were kept on that very highest shelf in the pantry: epsom salts, a huge bottle of liniment (bought from the Raleigh peddler in his horse-drawn van), occasionally turpentine, camphor oil, often castor oil, and always Corona Woolfat, whose metal container was so sturdily constructed as to leave a child without hope that it might be broken by accident.

My Aunt Eunice, who took me to raise when I was 6 years old, was convinced that Corona Woolfat was miraculous. She smeared it on everything from corns to acne. It was so foul-smelling that she left the windows open when it was applied, and its nasty consistency defied genteel comparison. I battled harder to avoid it than I ever did over castor oil. She had to send away for it, and when it was no longer available, she was heartbroken, while I silently rejoiced.

There was one other resource which my aunt often used. To Aunt Eunice, religion was a great part of life. After she had done everything that was humanly possible with the knowledge she had, the rest she left in God's hands.

I never knew any children in our community who were vaccinated. When the danger of smallpox was rumored, every child wore a hunk of asafetida in a bag on a string around the neck. It had a powerfully fetid odor, and it must have taken a stouthearted teacher to stay in a roomful of children so adorned on a winter day. But I never minded the odor as much as some people did. I had been conditioned by Corona Woolfat!

Aunt Eunice made most of our medicines from things found around the farm. She washed wounds with salt water or a weak solution of carbolic acid from the bottle kept for the livestock. Insect stings received a dab of mud or soda, whichever happened to be handiest. Burns were covered with lard or even butter if she was in a hurry. A boil might have a piece of fat bacon tied on it to draw it to a head. And, like most children of that day, I could count on being dosed with sulphur and molasses if, when spring came, my aunt thought I looked "puny."

Best of all was pennyroyal. Every fall Aunt Eunice hunted in the timber for the aromatic herb which she hung to dry in the back entry. When I developed sniffles, she filled a small wooden tub with hot water and while my feet soaked, she had me drink a steaming cup of pennyroyal tea. I can't recall particularly liking the flavor of the herb, but the cream and sugar in the cup were a delight.

If the cold went down into my chest, Aunt Eunice prepared a poultice. She began by roasting onions in the hot ashes and coals of the heating stove. When the onions were tender and piping hot, she folded them inside cotton flannel which she pinned to my nightie against my chest. They were delicious. I don't know if she suspected that I sneaked out some of the onions and ate them; if she did, she never rebuked me.

The last resort for a stubborn cold was the "sweat box." This granddaddy of the modern sauna had a trade name, but we knew it simply and appropriately as the sweat box. The adults seemed to find pleasure in it, so one cold winter evening I blissfully allowed Aunt Eunice to encase me, minus my clothes, inside those four oilcloth-covered frames. As she snapped the cover around my neck, I wriggled with anticipation. Soon I wriggled for another reason.

I sat on a small wooden stool under which there burned an alcohol lamp. For a while it was delightful, but when sweat began to ooze out of my pores, I

decided I'd had all I wanted and let everyone know it. They paid no attention to my protests; my set time for baking had not elapsed.

I realized I had made an awful mistake. Sweat rolled down my face in earnest, but I couldn't wipe it off because my arms were imprisoned beneath the cover. I howled in vain.

Then I became overwhelmingly aware that the stool was getting hot. I felt sure my bare bottom was going to be burned to a crisp. By this time Aunt Eunice was so hardened to my yelling that an eternity of minutes passed before she was persuaded to let me out.

The year of the great flu epidemic was frightening. One of my cousins died, as did many other people we knew. Our family stayed at home as much as possible, but sometimes it

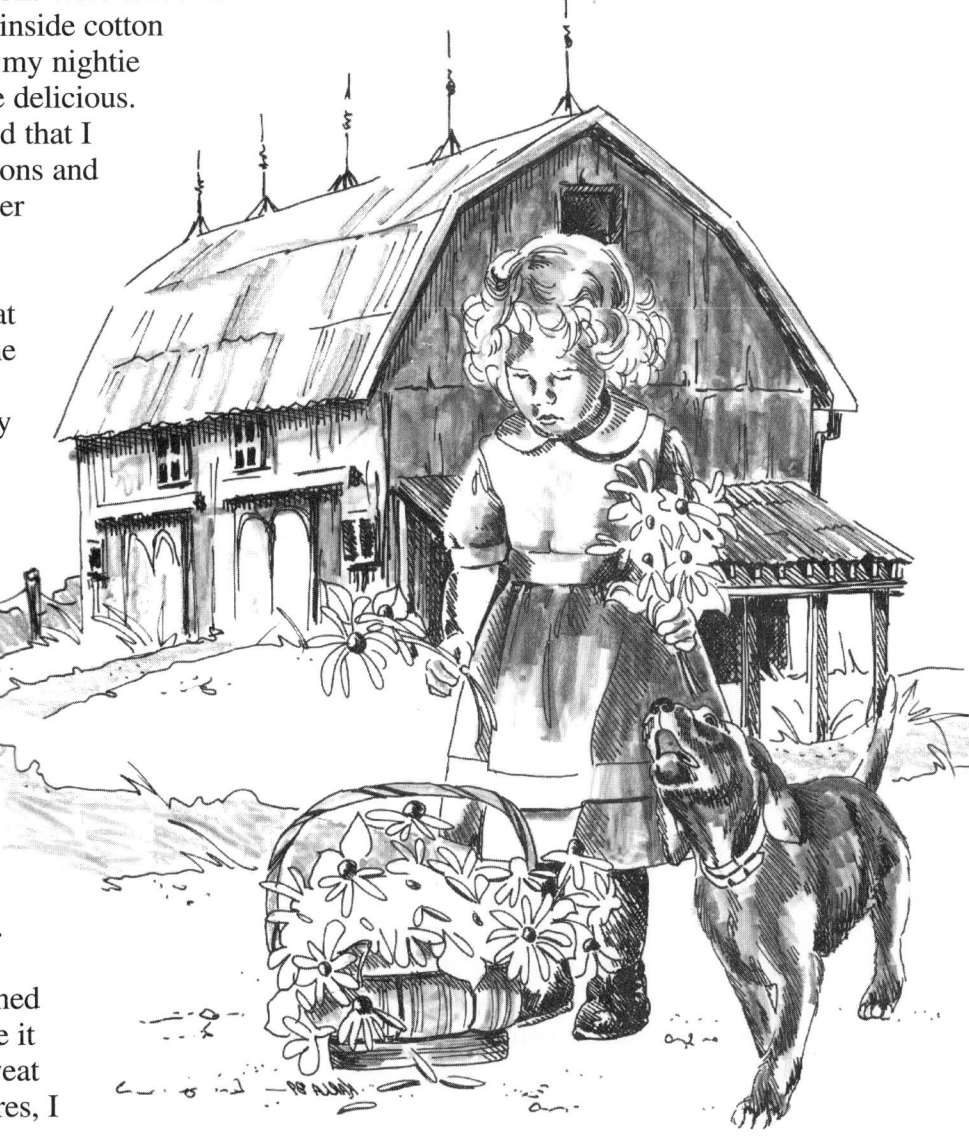

was necessary to go to town. The flu was thought to be harder on older people, so my sister and I drove the buggy to town, wearing masks of cheesecloth over our nose and mouth.

I did not get the flu but I was not as fortunate in escaping the common childhood diseases; I had them all, but fortunately for me, only one at a time. Whooping cough, diphtheria and scarlet fever— any one of them could have been fatal but I survived.

Diphtheria, however, almost got me. My aunt called the doctor, for I had become delirious. This was the first time I had ever seen a doctor, but I was too ill to be frightened by the stranger with the ominous black bag which he set on a chair at my bedside. He checked me over, listened to my labored breathing and shook his head.

"Membranous croup," he told my aunt, "and very bad." The mucous collecting in my throat was choking me. He didn't know how to get rid of it, but a croup kettle might make it easier for me to breathe, he said.

Aunt Eunice devised a croup kettle using camphor oil in hot water, but it did little good. I fought for every breath. Then one evening, my aunt, unable to bear watching my struggles, bent me over her lap, reached her fingers down into my throat, and pulled out a hard core of mucous. At last I was able to breathe and on the way to recovery.

The county health department quarantined us when I had scarlet fever. The placard tacked beside our front door was enough to send every visitor hurrying away. No one in the family, including the hired man, could set foot outside our gate. Occasionally we hailed a passing neighbor who would bring some necessity from town for us. He always left it well outside our fence.

This confinement wore on everyone,

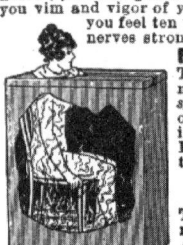
especially as I came through this illness much better than was to be expected and soon fretted to be outside. The whole family was eager to go for a ride in the shiny new Maxwell touring car we had recently purchased. The 40 days of quarantine expired, but the authorities delayed taking down our forbidding sign. Finally we couldn't stand it.

Our hired man was young and full of devilment, so I suppose the lark was his idea. He and Uncle Newt cut beards and mustaches from an old buffalo hide, donned wide-brimmed hats and backed the car out of the barn. The rest of us piled in and we sped about the countryside, causing all sorts of excitement.

The top of the car was down and we had muffled ourselves well against the brisk April breeze. Our neighbors thought they recognized the car, but not the occupants. One woman nearly tipped over in her rocker in her effort to get a better look. It was an exhilarating ride and raised our spirits immensely.

Finally a health department official came to take down the sign and fumigate with the formaldehyde which was supposed to get rid of any germs left lurking in the house. We took some food and blankets outside and sealed the door and windows as well as possible. Then the container of formaldehyde was lit. That night we slept in the barn and we cooked supper and breakfast over a bonfire. It was as good as a camping trip.

There was one other resource which my aunt often used, and I should not fail to mention it. To Aunt Eunice, religion was a great part of life. As I lay hovering near death, I became aware that she knelt beside my bed with head bowed. She had done everything that was humanly possible with the knowledge she had. The rest she left in God's hands. ◆

Old-Time Medicine Cures

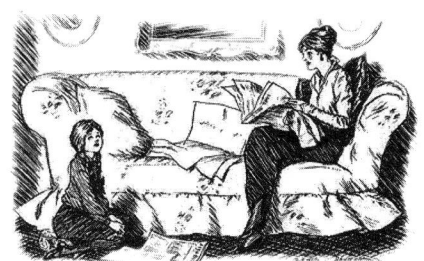

By Marlene Grant

The 'Little Giant' Cathartic, scarcely larger than mustard seeds, are sugar-coated. They remove the necessity of taking great, crude, drastic sickening pills, heretofore so much in use. As remedy for headache, dizziness, rush of blood to the head, tightness about the chest, bad taste of mouth, billious attacks, jaundice, pain in the kidneys, and internal fever, Dr. Pierce's Pleasant Purgative Pellets are unsurpassed."

So ran a January 1878 newspaper ad for these self-prescribed cure-all pills. In the 1800s, tonics, medicine and home concoctions were abundant as remedies for all known illnesses, and a few invented maladies as well. Sparsely settled communities and isolated cabins led people to depend on self-medication. Newspapers were filled with ads for tonics, pills and self-help books which would create good health and solve marital problems. In 1856, one pharmacist stated, "The chief mission appeared to be to open men's purses by opening their bowels." The non-prescription medical cures and advice business was booming in the 1800s because many people believed that one elixir could cure many illnesses.

Carter's Little Liver Pills was one of the many "liver invigorators" advertised to solve several medical problems. These liver energizers claimed to purify the blood, regulate the bowels, aid in digestion, and prevent headaches and seasickness, to name a few. It was years before Carter dropped "liver" from the pills.

Cancer cures also were meant to cure other ailments. Clay used to make red brick was used to cure tumors and rheumatism. After the clay dried, it was sieved and mixed in a jar with hot water until it became like putty. A half-inch of the mixture was spread on the affected part which was covered with light brown paper and bandaged for several hours.

Many cures were plant-based. John Wesley, among others, believed that God had provided a plant cure for every ailment. Many plants were known to be useful in alleviating certain symptoms; using willow bark to relieve pain, for instance. Today scientists know that willow bark contains salicin, a substance related to the salicylates used to make aspirin.

Lemons were widely used. They were supposed to correct billious-

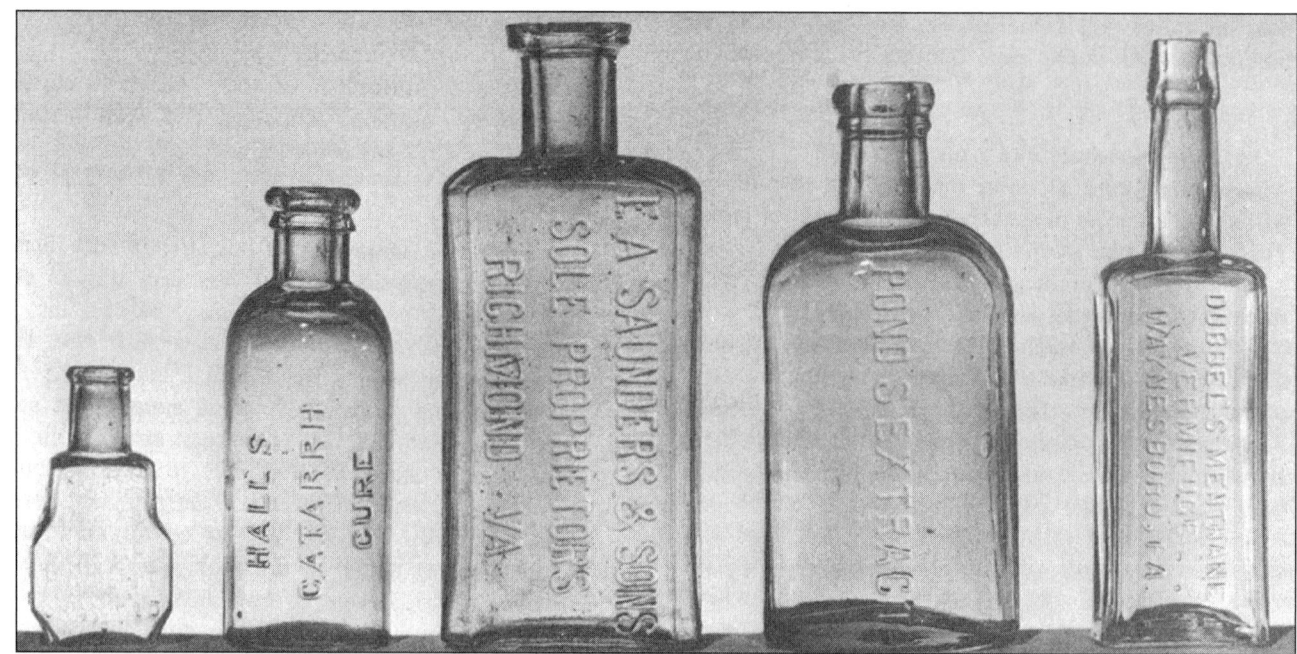

ness, worms and skin complaints. Gums were rubbed daily with lemon juice to keep them healthy. Neuralgia was thought to be cured by rubbing with a lemon. It was also used to cure warts and dandruff. Mixed with unsweetened hot, strong, black tea or coffee, it was used as a fever cure.

Medical books containing recipes for these and other cures were very popular because doctors were not readily available. One such book was written by Dr. Alvin Wood Chase in 1874. Chase gives some simple remedies, as well as some more complicated ones. For example, a sore-throat remedy of hot tea gargle was made with alum and honey dissolved in sage tea. A piece of borax as large as a pea was suggested as a cure for hoarseness. The best cure for nosebleeds was the vigorous chewing motion of the jaws which was believed to stop the blood flow; a child with a nosebleed was given a wad of paper and told to chew it hard.

A simple cure for heart palpitations was to hold one's breath repeatedly, and for as long as possible. It was hoped that this would keep the blood from absorbing oxygen as it passed through the lungs. Without blood passing quickly to the heart the excessive action would diminish.

Vomiting was also simple to cure, with kitchen ingredients readily at hand. Black pepper, salt, vinegar and hot water were mixed and taken every 10–15 minutes.

For sickness in general, beef tea was highly recommended. Beef was cut into small bits with no fat, then put into a bottle with cold water and corked. The bottle was set in a pan of cold water which was placed on the stove and allowed to come to the boiling point. Then the heat was reduced, and the water in the pan kept near the boiling point for 2 hours. The mixture was strained and the juices pressed out and seasoned with salt, pepper, and mace or nutmeg. Raw beef was also used as a cure for diarrhea.

Sex tonics reminiscent of some pills offered today in magazines were also touted by Chase and the newspapers. If these tonics failed, there were manuals which could be bought through the mail; naturally they arrived in a plain wrapper. These promised to restore virility without medicine. But Chase suggested that men make their own tonic pill, following this recipe: Strychnine, 3 grams; sulphate of quinine, 120 grams; iron by hydrogen, 120 grams; mix thoroughly and make into 240 pills. Take 1 pill every 6 hours during the day. After the system becomes used to them, take 1 every 4 hours. Dr. Chase remarked, however, that "the quinine should be doubled because he felt it would increase the tonic power of the pill."

A magic tonic for "weak and debilitated females" was recommended by Dr. Chase's wife. The recipe called for 4 ounces each of red Peruvian bark, prickly ash bark and poplar root bark; cinnamon bark, 1 ounce; cloves, ½ ounce; and whisky and clear worked cider, each 2 quarts. The bark was to be ground coarsely and put into the jug with the spirits and cider. The mixture was shaken daily for 10 days. The sediments were strained and the brew was poured into a wine glass after each meal. Dr. Chase enjoyed this drink himself.

The remedies of yesterday may sound dangerous to us. But the big business of self-prescribed medicine didn't fade with the 19th century. Medicine, pills, vitamin cures and self-help manuals abound. Now, however, several remedies may exist for one medical problem, as opposed to one remedy for several maladies, as in the past. ◆

The remedies of yesterday may sound dangerous to us. But the big business of self-prescribed medicine didn't fade with the 19th century.

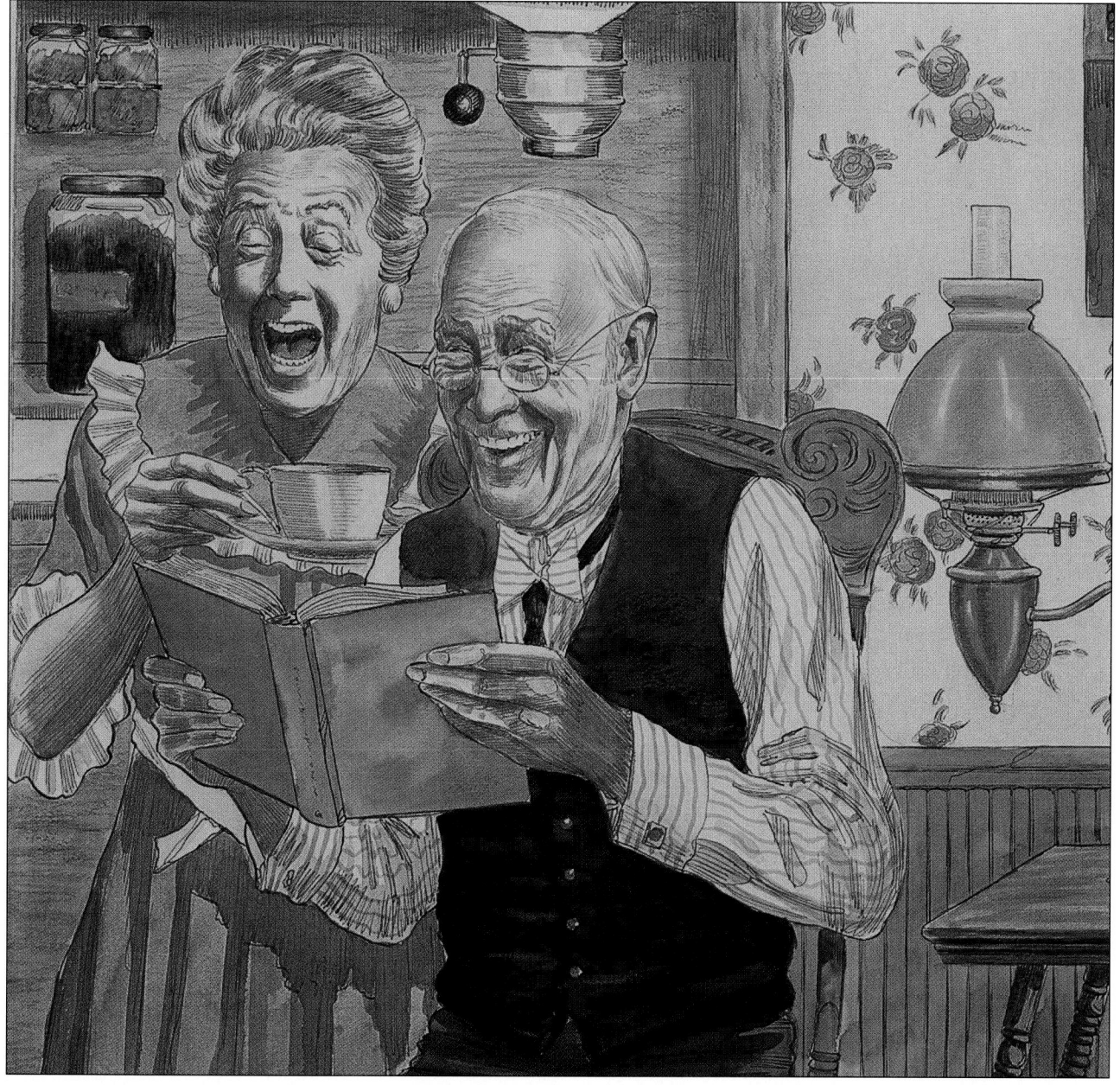

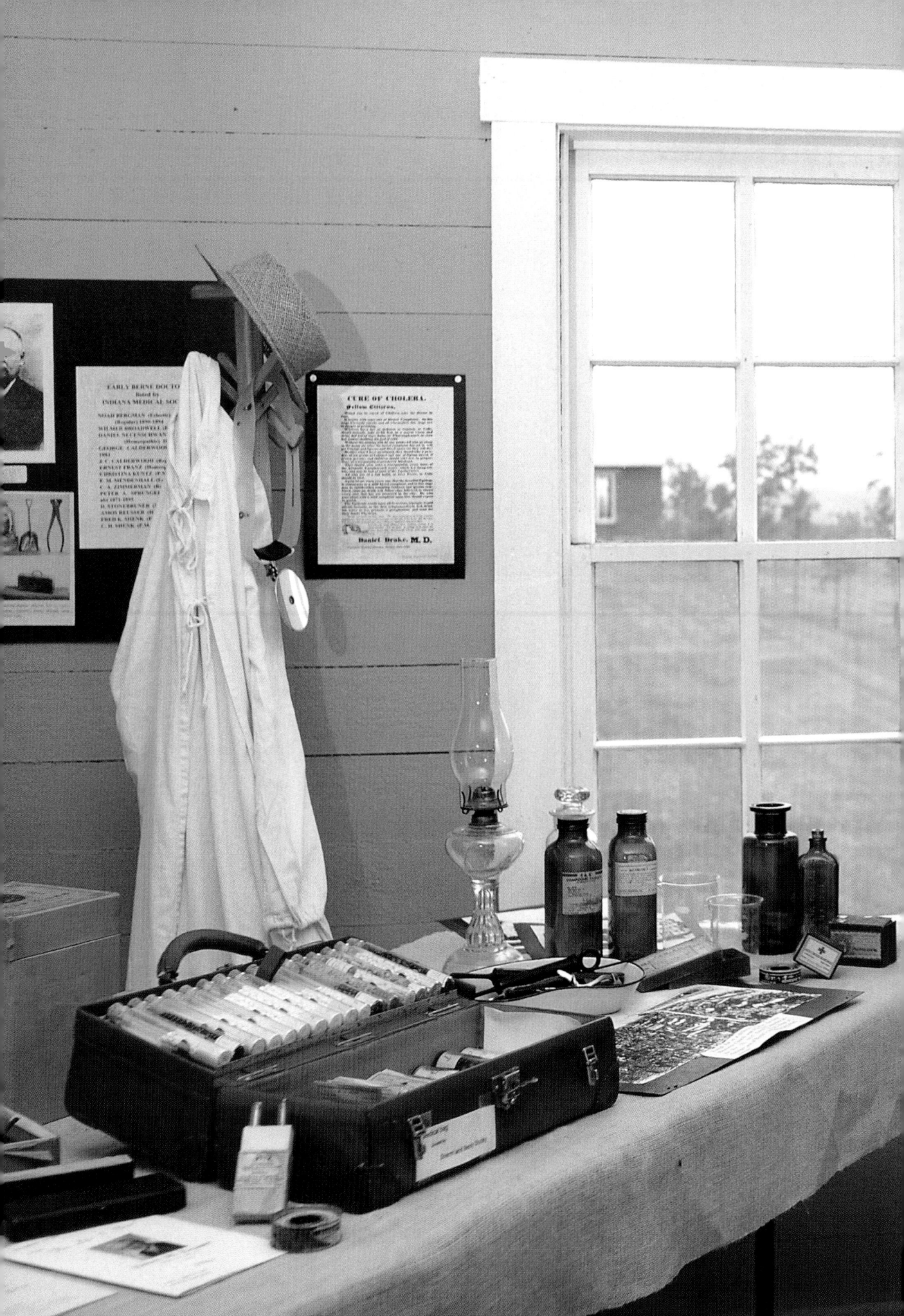

Chapter 5

COUNTRY DOCTOR, A FAMILY FRIEND

Country doctors were more than just physicians. They were friends. They were confidants. They were neighbors.

Doc Evans was one of the last country doctors in my Ozark Mountains. He arrived by train when there was no other easy way into the southern Missouri Ozarks. He spent the rest of his life treating the hill folk, their children and their grandchildren.

He provided all the professional health care we needed from cradle to grave. Oh, Doc Evans had an office in town, but that wasn't where you usually found him. Normally he was to be found headed out in his old jalopy for a remote farm on some emergency, whether real or imagined. House calls made up most of his doctoring, or at least that's the way it seemed. On the rare times we country kids saw a doctor, it was Doc Evans.

Home remedies would hardly be complete without stories of the country doctor—licensed and unlicensed—and other forms of home treatment. How could we have made it through the Good Old Days without them?

—*Ken Tate*

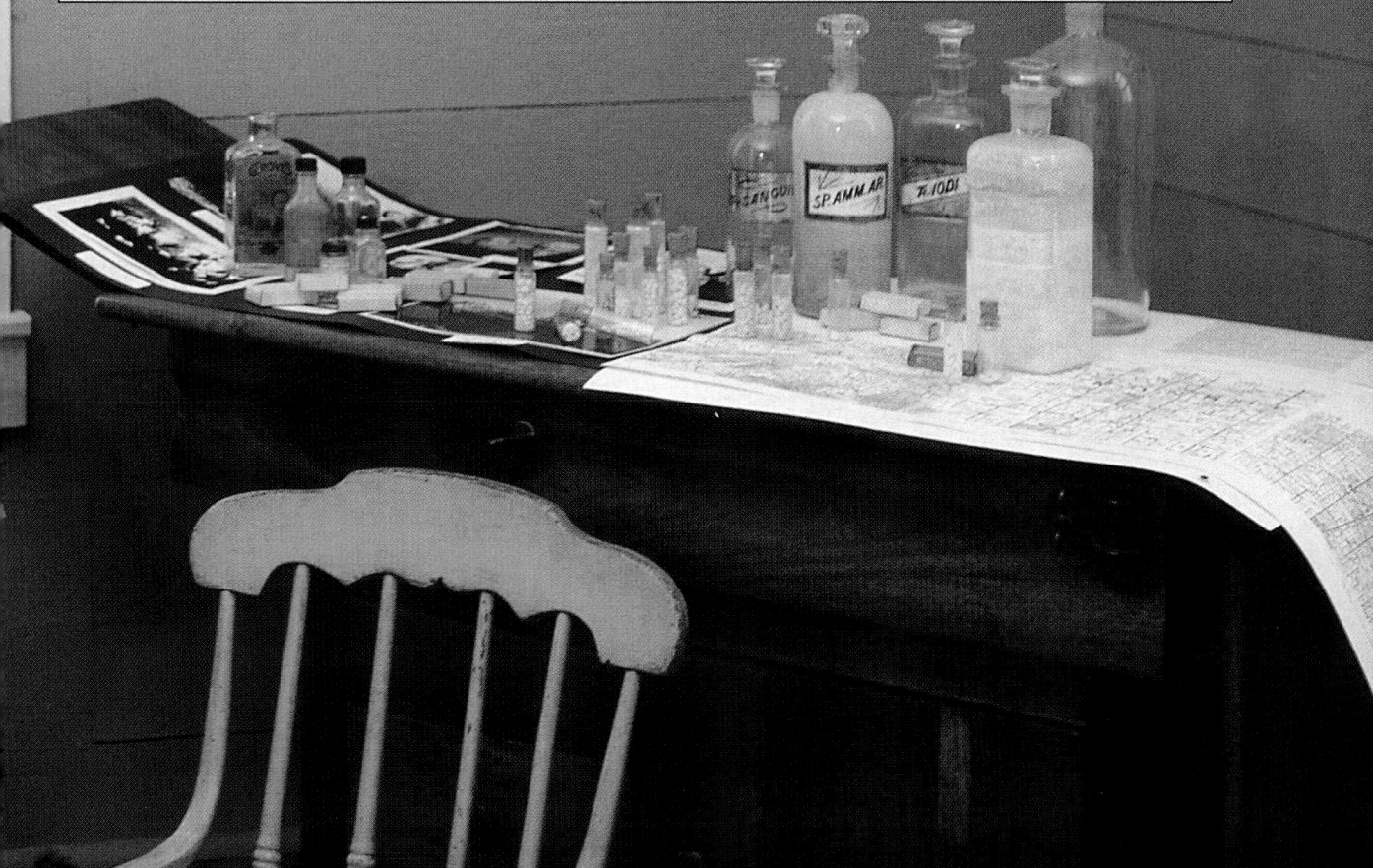

Country Doctor, A Family Friend

By Jewell Fitzhugh

Doctor, one of the mares kicked Mama in the stomach. She's hurt bad. We don't know what to do. Can you come quick to see about her?"

A girl's tear-laden, almost incoherent voice was calling old Dr. Hyden over a rural party line in a section of Northwest Arkansas in the late summer of 1917.

Reassured by the doctor's kindly tone and the promise to be on his way immediately, the girl hung up the receiver on the old-fashioned box telephone and returned to her mother's bedside, where the five anxious and fearful younger children were huddled.

How well I remember. I was the girl. Papa had died almost two months earlier, and now to have something happen to Mama brought terror to my heart.

I had been left at the house to wash the breakfast dishes and look after the younger children while Mama and Henley, my 10-year-old brother, went to the barn to do the feeding.

Only a few minutes had passed when Henley burst into the kitchen, white-faced and wide-eyed. "Hurry! Old Dolly kicked Mama. She can't get up."

Terror-stricken, we ran to the barn lot as fast as our legs could carry us and helped Mama to stand. Somehow, between us, and with her helping as much as she could, all the while telling us not to be afraid, we got her to the house and to bed.

Our Cousin Emma, overhearing my call on the party line to the doctor, soon arrived in her buggy. Minutes later old Dr. Hyden was getting out of his rig and hitching his horse to a tree near the front gate. To have present two ministering angels, the doctor and Cousin Em, somewhat relieved our fears.

> *Reassured by the doctor's kindly tone and the promise to be on his way immediately, the girl returned to her mother's bedside.*

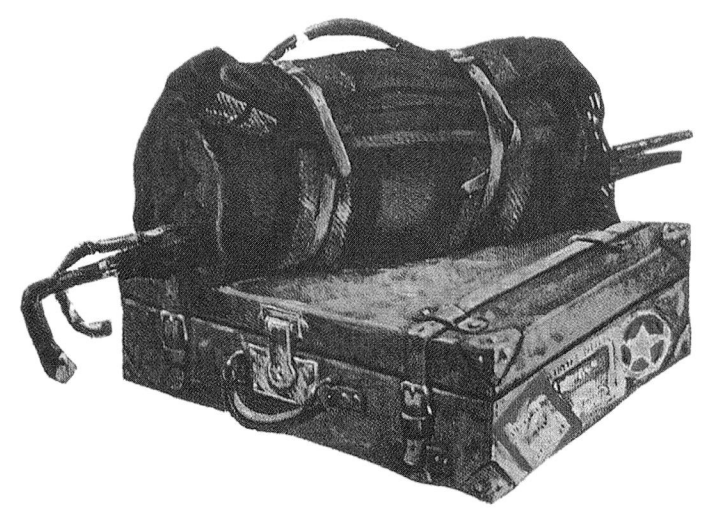

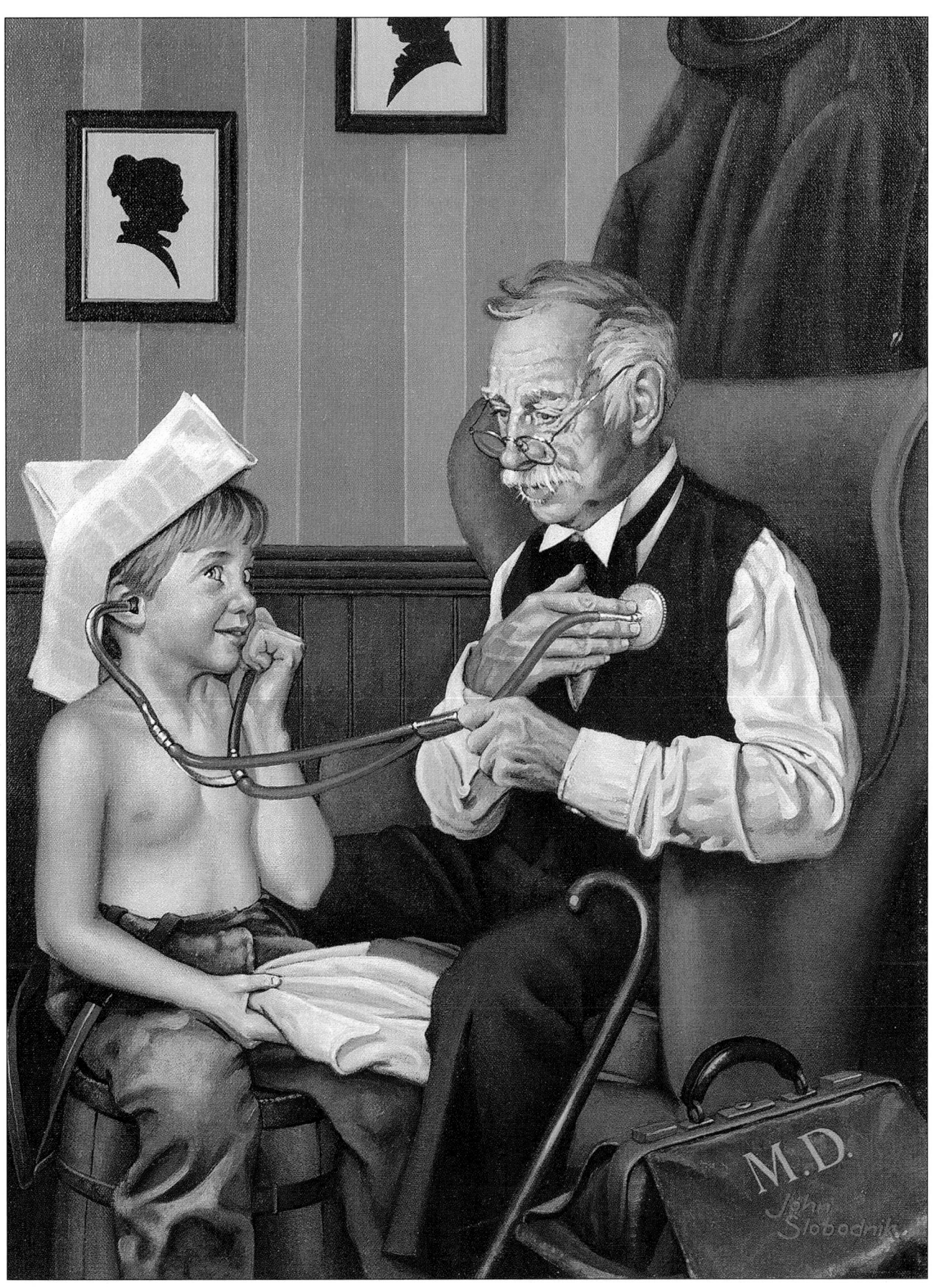

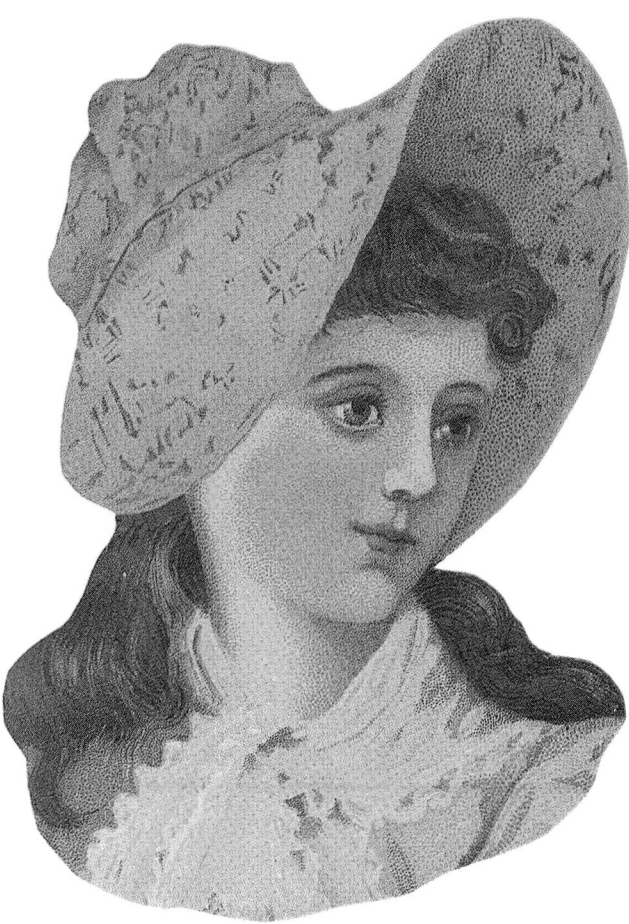

Papa had died almost two months earlier, and now to have something happen to Mama brought terror to my heart.

After examining Mama carefully, the doctor decided she was not seriously injured. Then he gave her some medicine from his black bag and told her to rest in bed for a day or two. Also, he told us to call him in case she didn't feel better the next day.

As I remember, he did not seem the least bit hurried, but talked and laughed with us. To us children he seemed terribly old—he even called our mother "child"—but we knew he was our friend. We could always depend upon him. When he left, we were not the disconsolate little brood that he found on his arrival.

An era of life vanished with the passing of the country doctor, the general practitioner,

subject to call 24 hours a day. In all kinds of weather, over all kinds of roads, he made his way to the most remote cottages and cabins to do what he could to alleviate human suffering. Pioneer doctors made their wide rounds on horseback, carrying their blue mass pills and other essentials in saddlebags. The earliest doctors that I can remember, before the advent of automobiles, traveled in one-horse buggies or light two-wheeled carts, called "jumpers." Come sleet or snow, wind, hail or high water, the doctor made his rounds to minister to pain-wracked patients, set a broken limb, or deliver a baby.

Sometimes the night was dark and cold. Stinging sleet and frozen roads caused the faithful old buggy horse to step carefully. The doctor was usually on his way to a remote farmhouse. His leather-gloved hands held frozen checklines. His little black medicine bag was under the dashboard beside his half-frozen feet. Sometimes the doctor's wife heated two bricks which she carefully wrapped and placed under the dashboard to keep his feet warm.

A doctor's wife was his main standby, aiding him not only by making home a happy place for him when he had time to enjoy the comforts of home, but also by ministering to persons who came to the house when he was away.

Many of the old-time country doctors had their offices in their homes, though some had tiny offices apart in crossroad villages. I am thinking particularly of an elderly doctor in a small country town in which I was teaching in the 1920s. His cubbyhole of an office was operated without benefit of nurse, bookkeeper or receptionist, but it was always a relaxed, friendly and comfortable place. In 1924, this physician covered 217 miles in one day, seeing his patients in four counties.

During the Depression, he made the following report to the County Medical Association: "Twenty-five percent will pay in produce, as they can; and 50 percent of the people can't pay, so I don't even bother to put them on my books."

The country doctor officiated at the births of hundreds of babies, often having delivered the father, the mother and the children in the same family. He was not only physician, but also friend and confidant to the people for miles around. Little children loved him, not only for the peppermint sticks or drops he passed out from the black bag, but for the way he had of making them feel important. He was jovial and kind. If at times he appeared gruff, it was only to hide a deep emotion of sympathy or grief he felt for a fellow human being. The doctor's step on the front porch and the sound of his hearty laughter often made a patient feel better.

Many of the early doctors relied a great deal on roots and herbs, but most had been to medical school and kept up their studies through the reading of medical books and journals. Quinine, turpentine, compound cathartic pills, calomel, castor oil, and herbal compounds were standard medicines.

In the early days before laws pertaining to medicine were as strict as they are now, a few may have just "taken up doctoring" because they were bent in that direction. In fact, I once heard an old-timer tell of a person who gave his deceased doctor brother's license to practice medicine to a man across the mountain who had decided to "take up doctoring." This, however, was an isolated instance and not the common practice.

Before cars, X-rays, wonder drugs, clinics, hospitals, and medical equipment had been developed to their present state, babies were born at home, and surgical operations were performed on kitchen tables.

In my early teaching days, I was boarding in a home in which the head of the household had to have a leg amputated. The successful operation was performed by the local doctor on the dining table by the light of kerosene lamps.

The country doctor was on hand for almost every emergency. On one occasion our family doctor delivered premature triplets. There was only one baby garment in the house, so two of the babies had to be wrapped in bits of cloth found by some neighbor women who were there. The doctor made an incubator of quilts and hot bricks to give the three infants a start in life.

One of the best things I can remember about the country doctor in the time of my growing up was his kindness and concern for the individual.

A particular incident from childhood is stamped upon my mind. One of my little sisters had a summer complaint that had taken as its toll the lives of several babies and small children in the surrounding country. One afternoon my grief-stricken parents thought

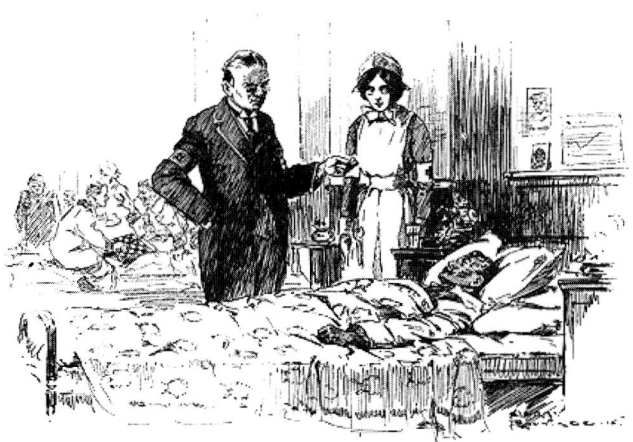

One afternoon my grief-stricken parents thought their child was dying. They sent for Doctor "Irving" who came immediately. Realizing the seriousness of the situation, he stayed by her bedside all night.

their child was dying. They sent for Doctor "Irving" who came immediately. Realizing the seriousness of the situation, he stayed by her bedside all night and until she showed signs of improvement the following day.

It was this and similar experiences that endeared the country doctor to all of us. Would that the doctors of today had more time for the individual. I am not ungrateful for the advances in medical knowledge and equipment and skill of the specialist; but I miss the personal touch, the warmth and friendliness of the old-time doctor, who not only knew me by name, but also knew my parents, grandparents and all our family background—our sorrows and joys. He was my friend. ◆

The Cold Cure

By J.C. Ellis

It was wintertime on that old dirt farm in Pennsylvania. It was the time of year for running noses and sore throats. In some places the snow drifted above the tops of the fences, and on the level it was a foot deep. In some places there were bare spots, and the ground was frozen as hard as glass.

I was 13 years old and big for my age. I was expected to do—and I did—my share of the chores around that farm barn. The cows were milked and the milk stored in cans before it was taken to the creamery. Jack and Jenny, our faithful team of mules, never failed to get the milk to the creamery on the bobsled. Other chores had to be taken care of and the horses had to be fed and watered. The chickens were fed and the eggs had to be hunted up to make sure none of them froze.

The hogs had to be fed a mixture of equal parts ground wheat and ground corn, mixed with sour buttermilk to the consistency of thick cream. The hogs were one of the main sources of income to us farmers, and we took great care to get them fattened up for butchering in as short a time as possible. Pigs born in February would weigh upwards of 300 pounds, dressed, in October. Our 130-acre farm never failed to produce enough food to fatten the hogs.

When I got up on this particularly wintry morning, I felt very queer. My throat was scratchy and sore, and on one side, my tonsils were swollen as big as a duck egg. My nose was runny and stuffed up so badly that I had to breathe through my mouth. There was no mistake

> *I was expected to do—and I did—my share of the chores around that farm barn. The cows were milked and the horses fed and watered. The chickens were fed and the eggs had to be hunted up to make sure none of them froze in the cold temperatures.*

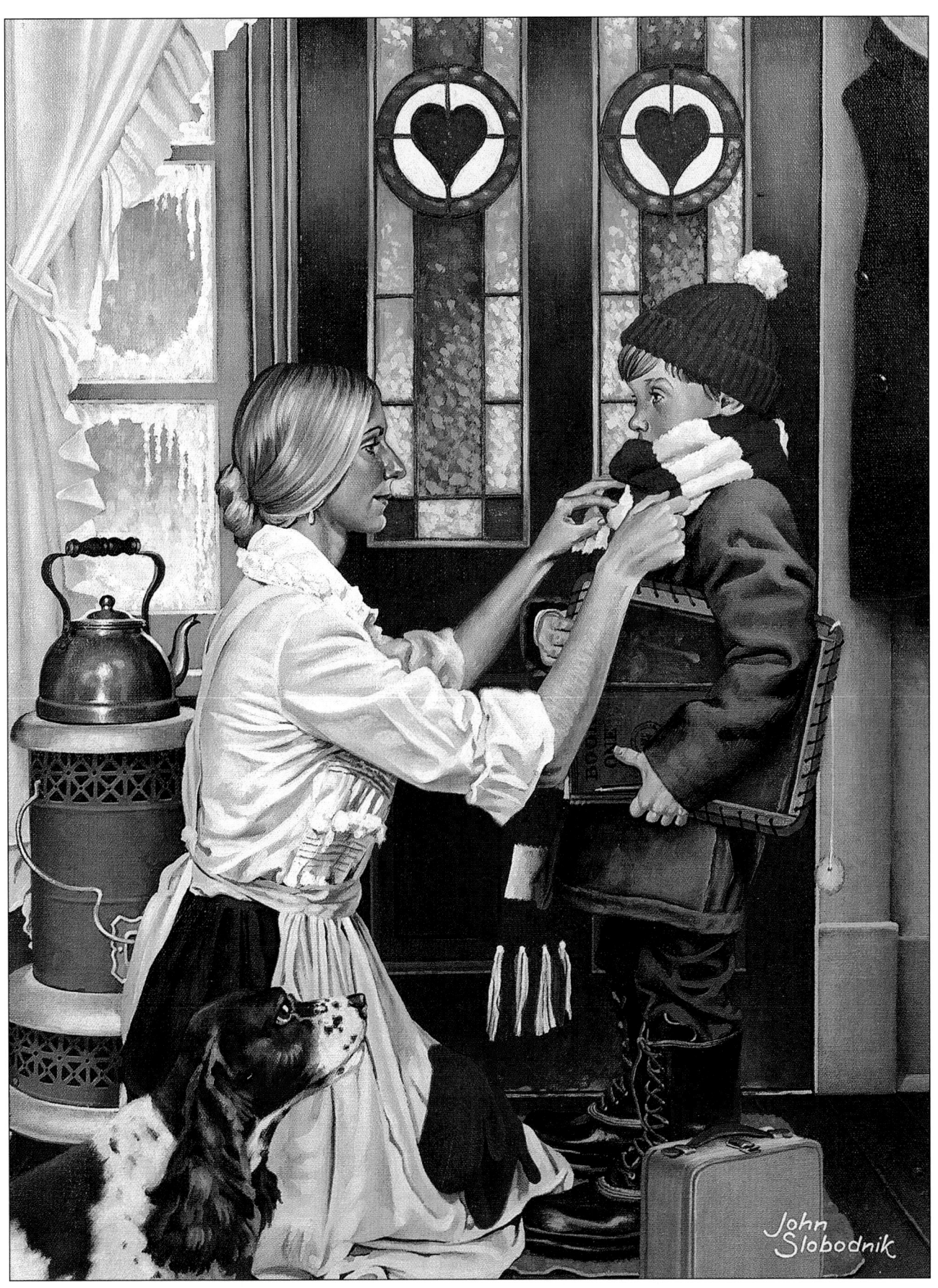

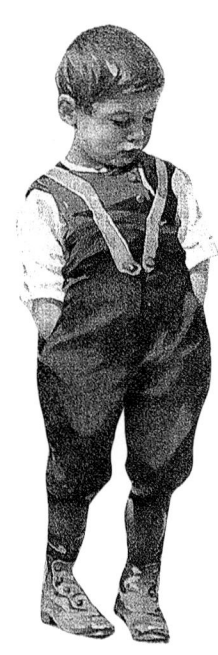

Just then Pop came in from the barn with two cans of milk. He took a good look at me and said, "As soon as we have breakfast, I'll show you how to get rid of that cold and that stiff neck."

about it—I had an old-fashioned cold.

When I came downstairs that morning I couldn't turn my head to the right or left. Mom was stirring the oatmeal, and as she looked at me, she exclaimed, "My goodness! What is wrong with you?"

I walked over to the window behind the stove and started to scrape off the thick frost so I could see the barn. But the snow was blowing so hard that I could hardly see it.

Mom came over and put her hand on my forehead. "You have a fever," she said. "I hope you are not getting the mumps. They will be coming in from the barn any minute now for breakfast, and I must hurry and have it ready." We usually had fried ham, scrambled eggs, oatmeal, toast and coffee, and sometimes fried mush as well.

Mom placed a piece of salt pork on the side of my throat which was more swollen. Then she wrapped some flannel around it and tied it with a stocking.

Just then Pop came in from the barn with two cans of milk. He took a good look at me and said, "As soon as we have breakfast, I'll show you how to get rid of that cold and that stiff neck."

Everyone seemed to enjoy breakfast but me. I couldn't eat a thing.

Mom said, "Get your sweater on, and a heavy coat and your felt boots. Pop is getting ready to go to the back woods and cut down trees, and you be ready."

Pop was a powerful, heavy-set man, as strong as an ox, and I don't ever remember seeing him with a cold. He got the crosscut saw and a couple of steel wedges and a big wooden maul.

"Josh, you get a shovel to shovel the snow, and bring the sandwiches your mother has made and we'll head for the back woods."

After a half-hour of trudging through the snowdrifts, we arrived at the northernmost tip of our farm. Pop selected a tall tree on one side on a small knoll and said, "Shovel the snow away from that tree, and a couple more trees while you are at it."

The sweat was running down my back from the trudge through the snow, but I felt comfortably warm.

Pop said, "Get ahold of the other end of that saw and we'll get started with this one." The tree was about 2 feet in diameter and it was a black oak, a hardwood, but the saw was sharp. It traveled right through that tree while Pop kept saying, "Faster, faster."

We were a little more than halfway through when the saw started to pinch as the wind made the tree sway. I was glad for a rest.

Pop started a steel wedge in the cutback of the saw. A couple of good whacks with that heavy maul and we were sawing again. Faster and faster we worked, and streams of sweat ran down my neck, but Pop kept saying, "Faster, faster."

By 11:30 a.m., the first tree was down and we ate the sandwiches Mom had sent along. Sandwiches never tasted so good, and I was enjoying a breathing spell.

It seemed no time at all before Pop was saying, "Let's go. Get ahold of that saw." By 3 o'clock, when the sun was beginning to go down, there were three big trees lying on the ground. Pop said, "Let's start for home."

I felt good, but tired. And best of all, the stiffness in my neck was gone, and the swelling had gone down, too.

That was more than 70 years ago. I can't remember just when or where that cold went, but it must be somewhere among those tall trees in the back woods of that old farm in Pennsylvania. ◆

The Country Doctor's Wife

By Helen Kitchell Evans

The country doctor's wife is brave,
Because she has to live
With him who dearly loves her,
Yet has so little time to give.

He wants to linger by her side
From morning until night,
But always there are patients
In their sad and painful plight.

Always there are calls
That come at dinnertime or dawn;
True to his profession,
He is up and soon has gone.

He will never have a fortune
For his loving wife to spend;
Now and then she may find time
For a visit with a friend.

But all in all, she has to make
A heavy sacrifice,
For Mrs. Country Doctor pays
Her part of Doctor's price.

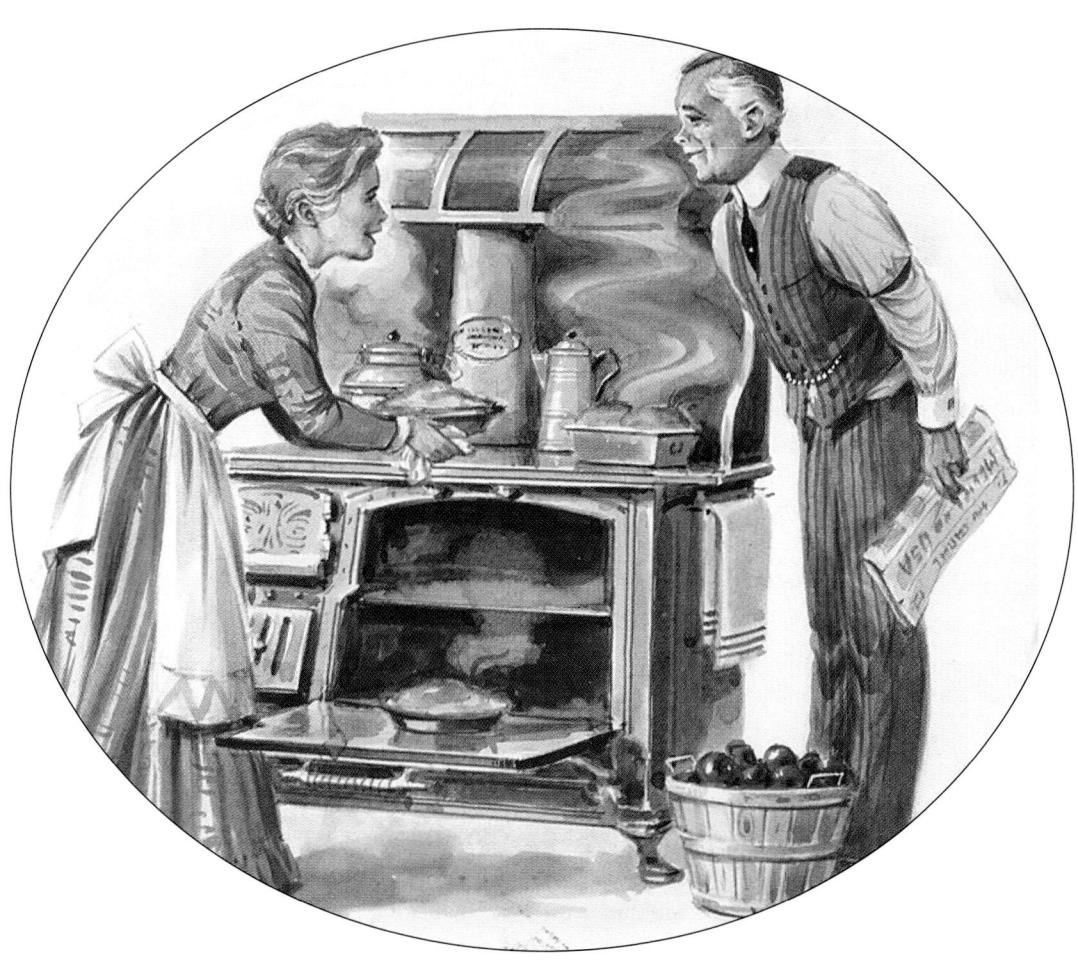

When I Was Young

By Bertha Holsinger

When I was young, I walked 4 miles to school after I cooked breakfast for my brothers and sisters and fixed their lunches. We were often late for school even though we ran most of the way. In the evening there were always dishes to be washed, floors to be swept, and wood to be chopped and carried in. By the time we were through we were too tired to get into too much trouble. When we hit the sack, we were "out" until morning.

It was really cold in winter. We had no thermal underwear, but I was happy to go to school with gunnysacks wrapped around my feet instead of overshoes. They were not much for looks but they provided good insulation against the cold.

At school our teacher would let us do some of our work huddled around the old potbellied stove. It had to be fed constantly to keep us warm.

Once my ears and toes froze on the way to school. The teacher washed them with kerosene to take the frost out and then rubbed them with snow to keep the heat down. My ears peeled for weeks, but they never dropped off.

One day, tromping through the deep snow, we all got so tired that we sat down out of the wind in a coulee to rest awhile. When I told the folks about it that night, they were furious and gave me an awful tongue-lashing. No matter how tired we got, they said, we must keep going.

Later we found out that some other children who had stopped to rest had fallen asleep and frozen to death. That's why our parents were so upset with us. I guess they usually had good reasons.

In the spring we walked through the nice mud after we had taken our shoes off. Sometimes we'd find wild garlic growing, and if we had a crust of bread left in our lunch bucket, it made a tasty afternoon snack. My mother said she could smell us coming if she couldn't hear us, but I can't remember being sick as much as kids are these days from overloading on popcorn, peanuts and pop.

The doctors were so far away that most of us never saw one; it took too long to get one. But castor oil was always in the house, as was liniment for our aches and pains. Aspirin was also around, but that was usually for Grandma's headache.

Once I had a broken arm and couldn't work in the field, so it was my job to take care of the young ones at home. One of my sisters was teething, and she was having convulsions and turning blue. I couldn't leave her to call my mother and I only had one good arm. But I picked her up and ran across the field with her under my sound arm to where my mother was.

A doctor was called. He cut her gums because her teeth wouldn't come through. The doctor said it was a terrible ordeal that the child had just gone through, as she needed rest and quiet. But she survived, and is now a grandma herself—and she's close to the doctor if she needs him. ◆

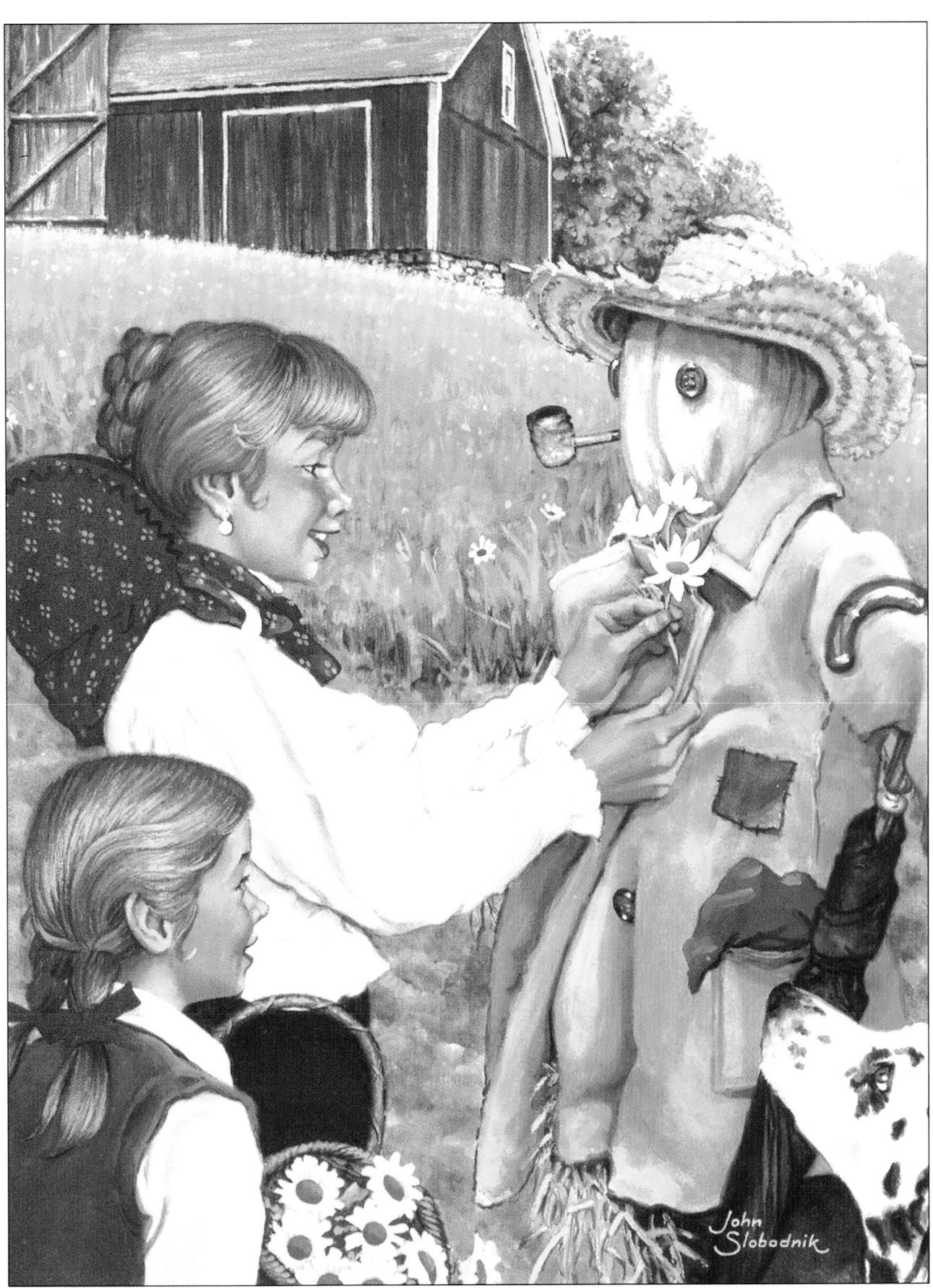

John Slobodnik

A Chain of Good Runners

By Mrs. B.M. Walker

My grandparents, Mr. and Mrs. Wellington McCurdy, took a homestead in the 1870s in north central Kansas. My mom was about 13 at the time.

They settled in Jewell County, Kans., near the town of Reubens. Today, I think Reubens is just four corners of the road—or at least it was the last time I was there; it may be covered by the lake that was put in a few years ago.

However, at the time Grandpa and Grandma lived there, Reubens was quite a flourishing little village with a mill, a store or two, a blacksmith shop, and even a doctor and lawyer.

Grandpa's place was 3 or 4 miles from Reubens, and a mile or so farther on lived another family—I'll call them the Does, as I can't recall their name. There were Mr. and Mrs. Doe, their son of about 10 or 11, their daughter who was a year or two younger, and Mr. Doe's elderly father.

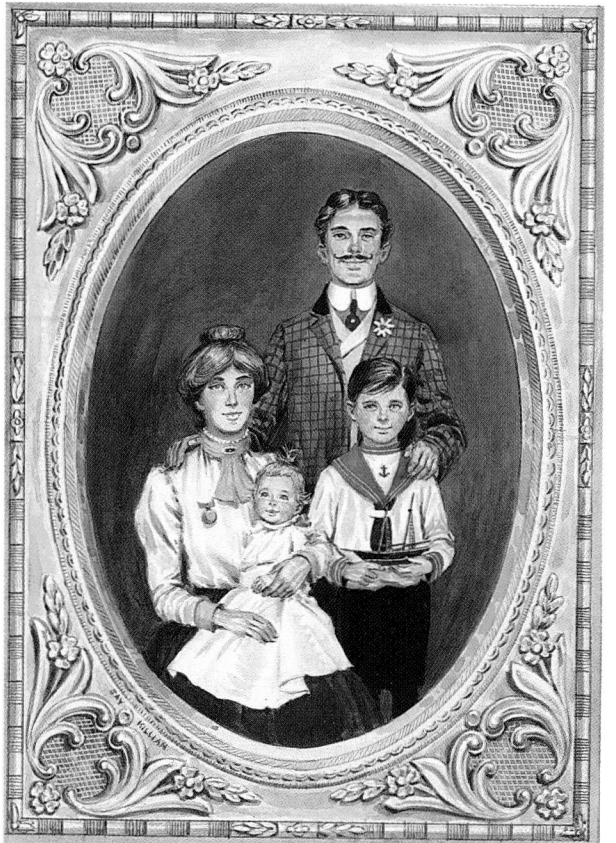

One morning Grandpa and Grandma went to see a neighbor who lived about halfway between their place and the village. Mom and her two younger brothers stayed at home, as their parents intended to return home soon. In those days people walked more, and my grandparents had walked to their neighbors' home.

About midmorning, Mom looked out to see the elder Mr. Doe running toward the house, gasping. Knowing it must be an emergency of some sort, she ran out to meet him. He panted out the question, "Where is your father?"

When she told him that her parents had gone to see their neighbors he said, "Quick, girl, run as fast as you can and tell your father to run on to Reubens for the doctor. My grandson has been bitten by a rattlesnake. I've run all the way here. I can't go any farther."

So Mom started running to the neighbors'. Fortunately she was an active girl, and she was used to running and walking. She arrived at the place where her father was visiting, told him, and immediately he took off at a dead run for the little village. Fortunately, the doctor was in his office, and also fortunately, his horse was fresh and was a fast traveler, so there was little delay in the return trip.

The Doe children had been pulling weeds to feed to the pigs, and a snake had struck the boy on the hand, between the middle fingers. The remedy the doctor used was this: A chicken was killed and speedily torn open, and the hand was encased in the body. As soon as the body cooled, another chicken was killed and used.

The boy recovered, although his arm was badly swollen for some time, and he was a very sick youngster for quite a while. But thanks to a chain of good runners, his life was saved. ◆

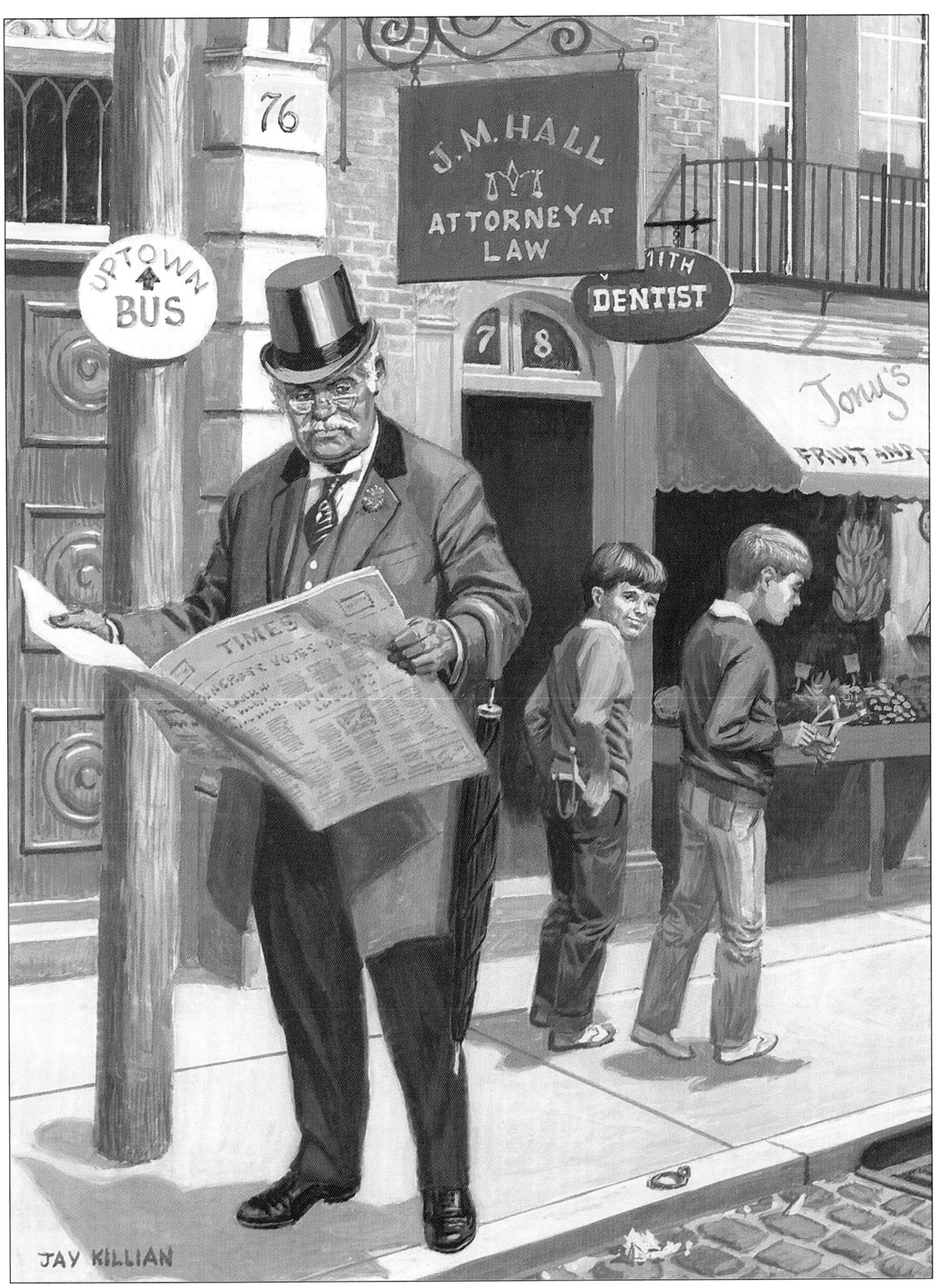

JAY KILLIAN

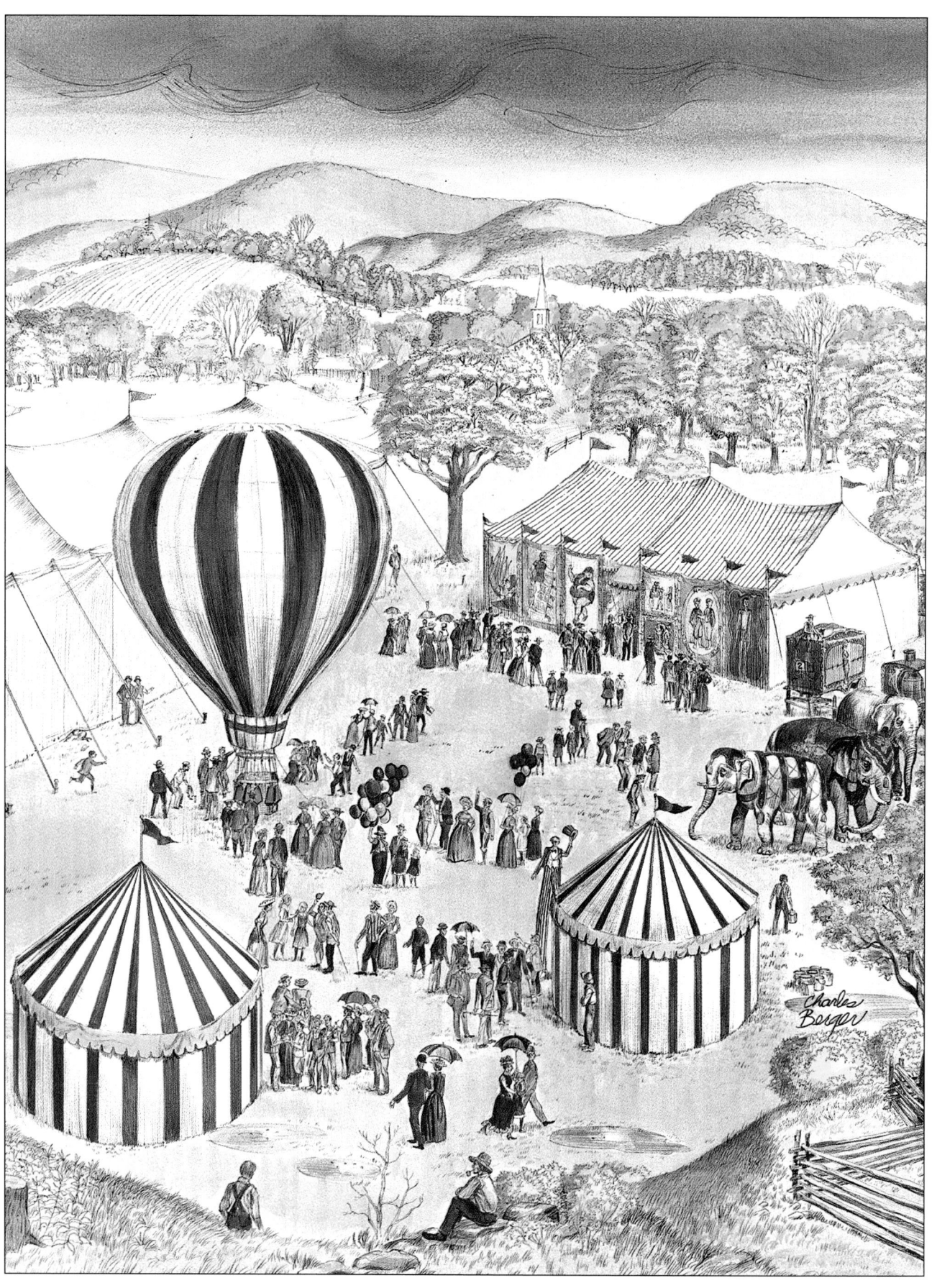

Caring for Ourselves

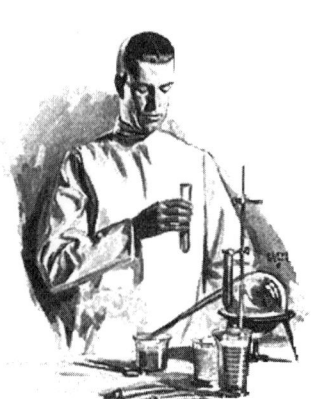

By Marjorie Covalt Yokaitis

Some of the ways in which people cared for their illnesses and personal welfare in the good old days are laughable in the view of today's enlightened society. The way we care for ourselves medically speaking has been and always will be an important aspect of life.

In the 1920s, as a child, I told an elderly neighbor that our family bathed daily. She was horrified! She said it was an unhealthy practice; that daily bathing took strength from the body and oil from the skin. And she proceeded to tell my mother so.

Mother listened respectfully, but being the daughter of a doctor, she knew what was right. We continued to bathe daily, but I was admonished for telling family secrets (I always was the family blabbermouth).

My grandfather was a little country doctor who drove around the Hoosier countryside in a horse and buggy, treating his patients. Doctors were not paid much in those days, over 100 years ago. If it was cash, it was only a few cents. Usually he was paid with a pig, chickens, vegetables or perhaps a quilt. But since Grandfather had a wife and a large family, these items were no doubt welcome.

Grandfather must have been afire with the desire to become a doctor, for he left a wife and family to enter medical school at about the age of 40. He did so with a clear conscience because he had three strong sons to carry on the work on the farm where they lived.

Little was remembered about my grandmother because she died at an early age. Sadly, the kidney infection which killed her could have been easily cured today.

Mother remembered going into the woods with her father to gather medicinal plants from which he made pills for his patients. He ground the plants with a mortar and pestle and formed pills from the mixture.

My mother recalled the time she contracted pneumonia. Her mother was still alive then, and Grandmother made tiny pancakes, putting in the center of them the pills my grandfather had made. The quarter-size pancakes so fascinated Mother that she readily ate them—and the medicine. Mary Poppins' song *A Spoonful of Sugar (Helps the Medicine Go Down)* hadn't been written yet, but Grandmother knew

Now, with the Salk vaccine, parents need never fear that dread disease. I am proud to say that my own three sons were among the first in the United States to receive the vaccine.

the wisdom of those words. She may have been among the first unofficial "practical nurses." She often assisted her husband when necessary—in childbirth cases and other circumstances, as well.

In those days, a mixture of lard and turpentine was rubbed on the patient's chest to treat a chest cold.

Knowledge of medicine was so limited in those days that only the very strongest survived. As a result, there came a generation of healthy offspring.

I recall a few medical practices from my own childhood days. One particularly ghastly tasting remedy for colds was a mixture of coal oil and sugar. No one who ever had a dose could forget it. It was one time when sugar did not help!

Mother was very aware not only of the need for cleanliness, but for proper nutrition and plenty of rest. In the summertime, when other children were playing in the warm night air, I was called in promptly at 8:30 to prepare for bed. Many arguments ensued, but I was still called in. How I have blessed her through the years for her strict adherence to her health rules, because for the most part, I have enjoyed good health.

We were given a good dose of castor oil when necessary. How I complained about that! Even today "good old castor oil" (if you can call it "good") is still sometimes used. Having experienced this treatment recently before having X-rays, I can testify to the fact that it tastes as horrible today as it did when I was a child—and it leaves no doubt as to its effectiveness!

When my tonsils were removed, I didn't go to the hospital, but to my doctor's office. After the ether had worn off, I found myself in my little bed at home. Mother soothed my burning throat with a Popsicle which, I believe, was fairly new on the market.

As a child I heard little concerning polio, but it came to my attention rather sharply when I was about 15. It was the week of the county fair, a week all children looked forward to all year long.

Our church sponsored a dining hall on the fairgrounds. All women cooked or served food, so the children were admitted free. We spent the entire week at the fair, going home only to sleep. It was a week of pure pleasure. We

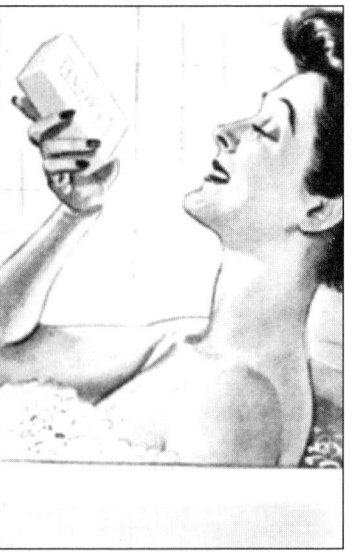

I told an elderly neighbor that our family bathed daily. She was horrified and said it was an unhealthy practice!

children rode all the rides and visited the side shows as long as our slim pocketbooks held out.

This particular fair week, Mother, my sister and I had just arrived at the dining hall when Mother received a phone call from my older brother, who had followed in his grandfather's footsteps to become a doctor. He told my mother that there were an alarming number of new cases of polio at the hospital. He told her to get my sister and me out of the fairgrounds and away from the crowds as soon as possible. She sent us home, posthaste.

During the ride home, my sister and I used every cuss word in our limited vocabulary to describe our brother. He was mean! He was an ogre! He had delighted in ruining our wonderful week of fun!

How could we teen-agers know the wisdom of his advice, and understand the suffering he might have spared us? Now, with the Salk vaccine, parents need never fear that dread disease. I am proud to say that my own three sons were among the first in the United States to receive the vaccine.

How far we have come in a little more than 100 years—from the little country doctor, gathering plants to treat his patients, to all of today's marvelous medical discoveries.

I believe that in the next 100 years much progress will be made in this area, and the world will be a better, decent place in which to live. You say I'm a cockeyed optimist? You bet! Care to join me? ◆

Battling Boils

By Patricia Misiuk

When I was a teen-ager, I pouted on bad hair days, struggled to conjugate Latin verbs, and smeared flesh-tinted goop over ever-present pimples. But nothing compared to my four-year bout with boils.

Yet, I survived, thanks to a chemical-free, environmentally friendly home remedy.

During the early 1950s, when milk came in narrow-necked glass containers, Mom enlisted the aid of an empty bottle as an alternative to lancing the boils.

She dunked a clean empty bottle into a large pot full of water and brought the "mixture" to a boil (no pun intended). Carefully removing the heated bottle, Mom placed it neck down on the skin surrounding the boil.

As the air inside the bottle cooled it contracted, forming a partial vacuum, and forcing the bacterial sludge and its afterbirth to erupt from the boil. The process was painless and complete. Needless to say, I welcomed the relief.

Fortunately, by the time plastic milk containers phased out their clear breakable counterparts, I stopped getting boils. ◆

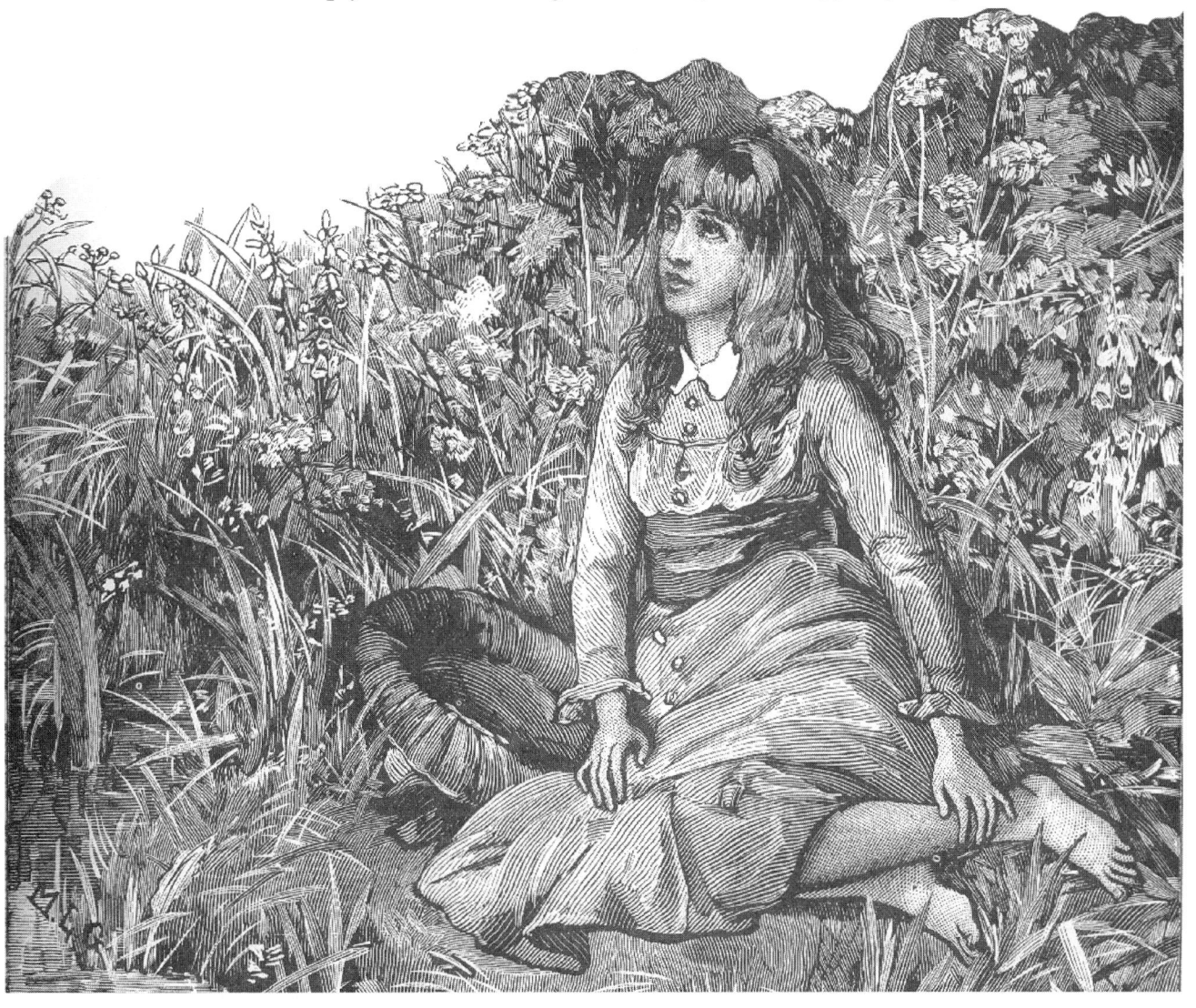

Early Day Doctoring

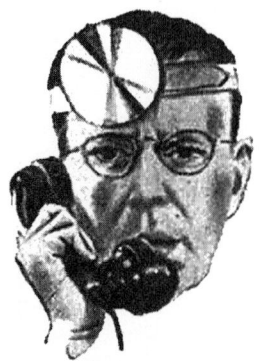

By Margaret Underwood

At first Mom thought she had spells of indigestion. Every once in awhile her right side would hurt for a couple of days. The pain would then ease back to mild discomfort.

Finally a day came when the pain was much worse. The nearest physician, Dr. Ingersoll of Ephrata, Wash., 12 miles from our town of Adrian, Wash., was summoned by phone, and he was definite in his diagnosis. "Mrs. Norman, you have acute appendicitis and must be operated on right away."

Mother was equally definite. "I won't go to any hospital, and that is that!"

Dad tried to convince her. "Pearl, the doctor says if your appendix bursts, you will get gangrene and die."

"I'm sorry, Frank, but I had enough of hospitals when my children were born. I would rather die than go to a hospital again."

"I guess her mind is made up, doctor. Is there any other way she can be helped?"

The doctor said reluctantly, "I have seen a few cases where the patient wasn't operated on, but I warn you, it is risky."

"Just tell us what to do, and we will do it."

"First, you will have to use ice packs on the painful area for several days. No solid food at all. She is to have doses of mineral oil each day and the juice of oranges."

The doctor's orders were carried out to the letter. It was a worrisome time for the family. Mom slept in a bed in the living room. Day after day ice packs were wrapped and applied to the feverish area of her right side.

The house seemed so different without Mom bustling about, making meals, doing washings, ironing, and the many tasks mothers seem to do that aren't noticed until they are left undone.

> *The doctor's orders were carried out to the letter. It was a worrisome time for the family. The house seemed so different without Mom bustling about, making meals, doing washings, ironing, and the many tasks mothers seem to do that aren't noticed until they are left undone.*

We four children—ages 7, 9, 10 and 11 years—had to learn to be more independent during this time. Father had always helped with household chores, so he kept things running more or less smoothly. We were warned to not pester our mother.

After the first week dragged by, Mom felt a little better and the doctor had to admit she seemed to be improving.

Once Mom was feeling better, it was a treat to be able to sit by her bed for a few minutes and just visit with her. Ordinarily it seemed she

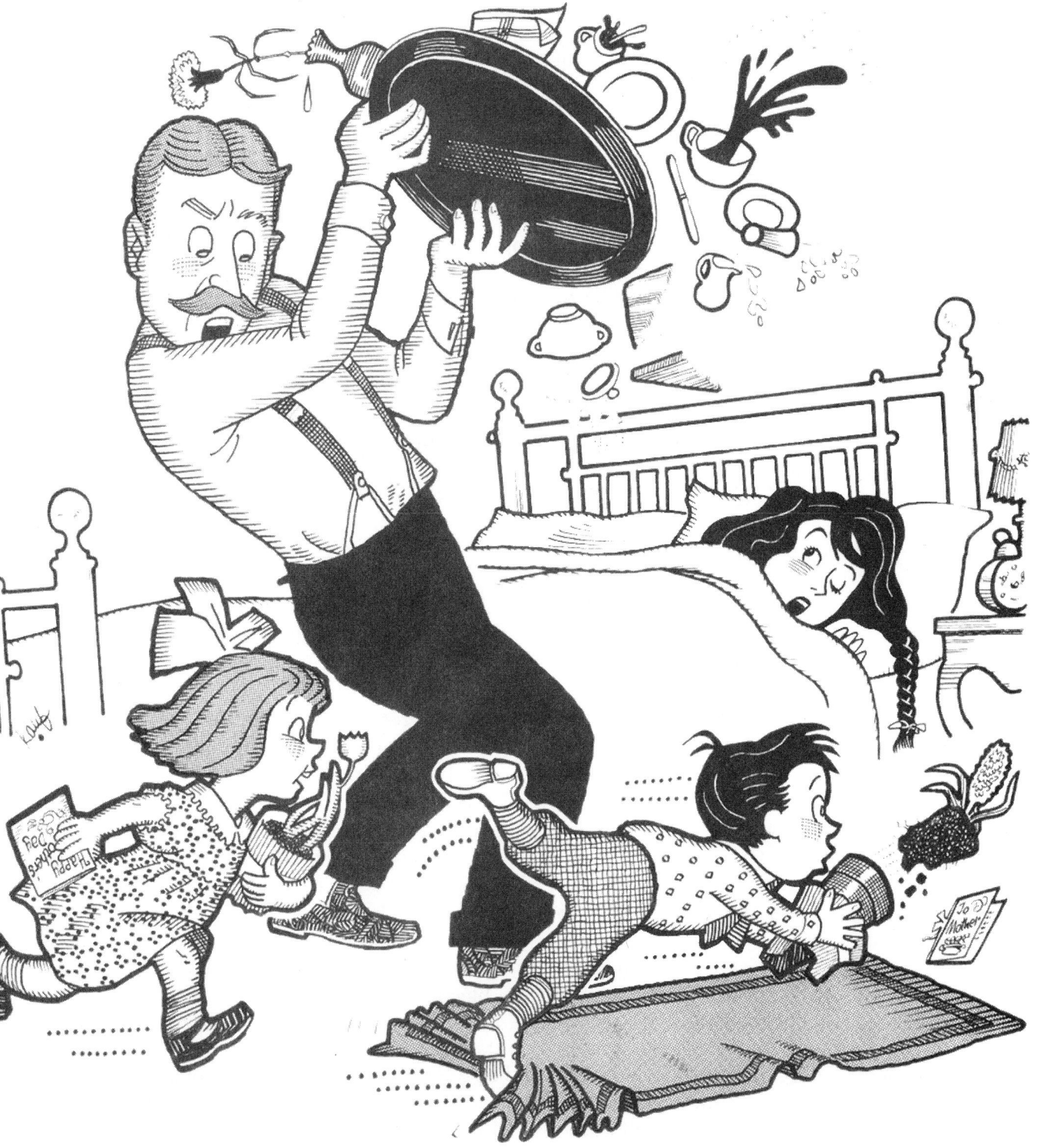

was too busy to just chat.

I was 9 years old that year, and remember yet confiding to Mom my most secret dream. It was a dream that someone would abandon a baby on our doorstep with a note that it was to be given to me. I was too near in age to my youngest sister to remember her as a baby, and to me a baby seemed like a toy that could be played with, then put down when I felt like doing something else. Mom must have smiled at my innocence.

Anyway, at the end of a long month, Mom was back on her feet and back to her busy routine. The living room was once more just a living room, and although she lived to be 87 years old, she never had trouble with her appendix again.

To understand how a later accident happened to me, you will have to picture a skinny, freckle-faced, red-haired girl-child sitting in an old, round washtub. I am shouting, "Mama, this bath water is cold!"

Mama answers from where she is working in the kitchen, "It is warm enough. Just scrub yourself and get out of the tub so Pearlie can bathe."

"No, Mama. Jane took too long to bathe, and the water is cold. I want a warm bath."

The water in the tub had been hand-pumped from the well in the back yard, heated in the wash boiler on the wood range, and dipped with a cooking kettle to pour in the tub. We had no bathroom, but the small storage room off the kitchen gave us privacy for summer bathing.

Sister Jane, being the oldest of we three girls, was given the privilege of the first use of the bath water. She may have finished her turn quickly enough, and I might have dawdled, but at all events the water had cooled.

"Please, Mama, couldn't I have some more hot water?"

"Oh, all right, Margie, the tea kettle is

Once in a while her faith in doctors would revive, and she would come back from her visit to him with a brown glass bottle of medicine guaranteed to work miracles. She would taste it and declare, "I know what is in this, but it isn't what I would use for what I've got."

boiling. I will bring in some water."

Mama hurried into the room carrying the heavy, cast aluminum kettle. "Now you get clear out of the tub. This water is boiling hot."

Bubbling with laughter, I got out of the tub except for one leg which was near the edge of the water. "You start pouring, and I will jump out," I teased.

Just as Mama started pouring the stream of boiling water, I jerked my foot upward. The bottom of the tub was soapy, and my leg slipped under the water gushing from the spout of the kettle. I shrieked with pain. Carrying me to a cot in the kitchen, Mama ran to the home of Rose Short across the street.

Rose was a calm, serene person, a good friend to have in emergencies. She said to Mom, "Get several potatoes and your grater."

As fast as she could work, Rose grated the raw potatoes and packed them around my leg.

As soon as the air couldn't reach the burn, the pain stopped as if by magic. The coldness of the potatoes kept the burn from going deeper into the tissues.

In a couple of days the leg developed huge blisters, but Mama used an ointment and kept the burn covered lightly with strips of soft, worn sheeting. In a few weeks the burn had healed with no scars.

Another time when we had to call our rough and ready Dr. Ingersoll was when my sister cut her ankle deeply on the edge of a metal can. The doctor was only called when there was no other choice and the gaping cut wouldn't stop bleeding.

The doctor was a heavy drinker, but never seemed to be so drunk that he forgot his doctoring skills. It took around an hour for the doctor to travel the 12 miles from Ephrata to Adrian, and the first order he gave was for a couple of strong people to hold the patient still while he sewed. This didn't seem to be in the days of pain-killing shots, or else he didn't believe in them. With my sister held down firmly by helpful neighbors, the doctor proceeded to slosh iodine into the open cut and stitch the wound while my sister's screams would have put a steam whistle to shame. The rest of us cringed in sympathetic terror with our hands over our ears.

I must grant the fact that the cut healed nicely without infection. It was also a perfect object lesson to the rest of us to watch our steps more carefully.

For some reason there were no broken bones in our family. None of the six members of the family had any broken bones. Maybe our diet rich in milk, butter and eggs and low in desserts gave us strong bones, or maybe we were all very cautious. After all, we sure didn't want to risk having to have a visit from our good Dr. Ingersoll.

Our Grandmother Jane was born in 1850 and grew up with a firm belief that any medicine that didn't taste horrible couldn't possibly cure any ailment. Mother, born in 1884, agreed with her mother-in-law in many of her ideas. They both trusted implicitly in castor oil, Epsom salts, quinine, sulphur and molasses, and the judicious application of Sloan's liniment.

Growing up, we had the benefit of mustard plasters, onion plasters, and smelly ointments guaranteed to "loosen our colds," but we lived anyway.

Grandmother Jane seldom ever saw the inside of a doctor's office. The thought of the $2 office fee, plus the 12-mile trip to Ephrata, generally made Grandmother decide to "wait a day or two and see if I get better." She generally did.

Once in a while her faith in doctors would revive, and she would come back from her visit to him with a brown glass bottle of medicine guaranteed to work miracles. We would watch her pull the cork from the bottle, wet a finger with a couple drops of the liquid and taste it. Smacking her lips a few times she would declare, "I know what is in this, but it isn't what I would use for what I've got."

Then she would store the bottle in her cupboard and proceed to get well without the help of the magic elixir concocted by the hard-working doctor. After all, she had successfully raised six children and that doctor probably didn't have as much experience as she did!

If a grandchild happened to pass by when Grandmother was checking the taste of the

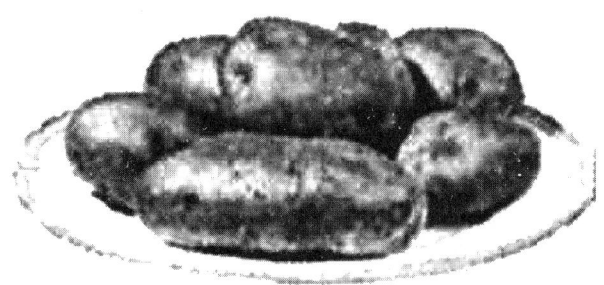

She said to Mom, "Get several potatoes and your grater." As fast as she could work, Rose grated the raw potatoes and packed them around my leg.

medicine, she would pour a little of the liquid into a spoon and insist the child drink it. She would say, "It will do you more good than it will me." We learned at an early age to disappear fast if Grandma had a bottle in her hand. Since she lived with us, maybe the medicine helped her get a little relief from four noisy, pesky grandchildren.

Grandmother died at the age of 82 when I was 10 years old. She never lived to hear of antibiotics and the many medicines that cure disease today. If she could walk down the aisles of a modern drugstore, she would no doubt pick up a bottle of medicine, unscrew the cap, taste a drop from a fingertip and declare, "I know just what is in this stuff, but it won't cure me." ◆

Winter's Woebegone Remedy

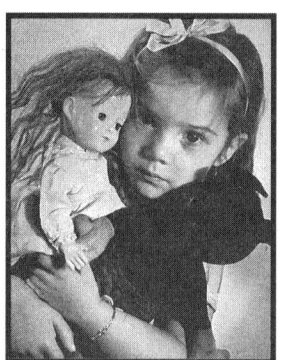

By DoraEllen Flint

Every spring, I think back to my grandmother and her various tonics. My fondest memory is of her sassafras tea. Evidently sassafras bark was unknown in western Montana, as my aunt who lived in Ohio would send my grandparents a package of it.

If I could convince Grandfather that I had been a real good girl, he gave me a cup of sassafras tea. Grandmother did not like the tea and thought sulfur and molasses was a much better tonic for growing children. "It puts more iron in your blood," she used to say. *Who needs iron?* I thought.

My brother and I learned that if we could feign a stomachache we would be given charcoal-and-pepsin tablets. Those black, gritty, mint-flavored tablets turned our tongues black. My brother discovered that they could be softened and we could smear them around our faces to make beards and mustaches. Mother never caught us, or you can rest assured that there would have been no more charcoal-and-pepsin tablets, regardless of how our stomachs ached.

My nemesis was wearing an asafetida bag. If you've not had the opportunity to smell its unusual aroma, you don't know how lucky you are. Asafetida is a resin obtained from an Asiatic plant of the parsley family. I can't fathom how a plant which is used so frequently in cooking and to enhance the appearance of a dinner plate could ever produce such a vile-smelling gum.

However, it wasn't the gum which smelled so bad, but the combination of herbs and spices which were kneaded into the gum. Some were ground cloves and ginger—but it was the garlic which gave longevity to the aroma!

I had to wear an asafetida bag during the winter of first grade. My grandmother insisted I would not get any childhood disease while I wore it, and she was absolutely correct. The odor was so terrible that no one wanted to be within 5 feet of me! How could anyone be exposed to disease while wearing an asafetida bag?

Grandma assured me I was fortunate to have one which looked like a pendant, as it was heart-shaped and crocheted of shaded lavender. She said that her children had had to wear asafetida bags made of flannel,

From the day after Thanksgiving until Good Friday, I had neither friends nor illnesses.

with strings sewn on for ties.

This didn't make me feel any better. I would have gladly given anyone the privilege of wearing it—if I could have found anyone who would come close enough. I tried desperately to untie it, but to no avail. (Grandma had probably tied it in a double knot.) So from the day after Thanksgiving until Good Friday, I had neither friends nor illnesses.

I think my mother, aunt and uncles probably suffered through the same ordeal—but back then, *all* the kids in their country school wore the smelly, terrible asafetida bags. However, I am sure that Grandma did not take into consid-

eration the fact that the school I attended was well-heated. She remembered how her children's schoolhouse was cold and drafty, heated only by a small "airtight" heater. (The parents furnished "their share" of wood and the older boys kept the wood box filled.)

Years later, Grandma admitted that the asafetida bag must have been a traumatic ordeal for a first-grader. I still remember vividly that awful smell; it took me years to muster up the courage to use garlic in cooking. My only salvation was knowing spring would come and I would once again have the pleasure of slowly sipping the wonderful sassafras tea. ◆

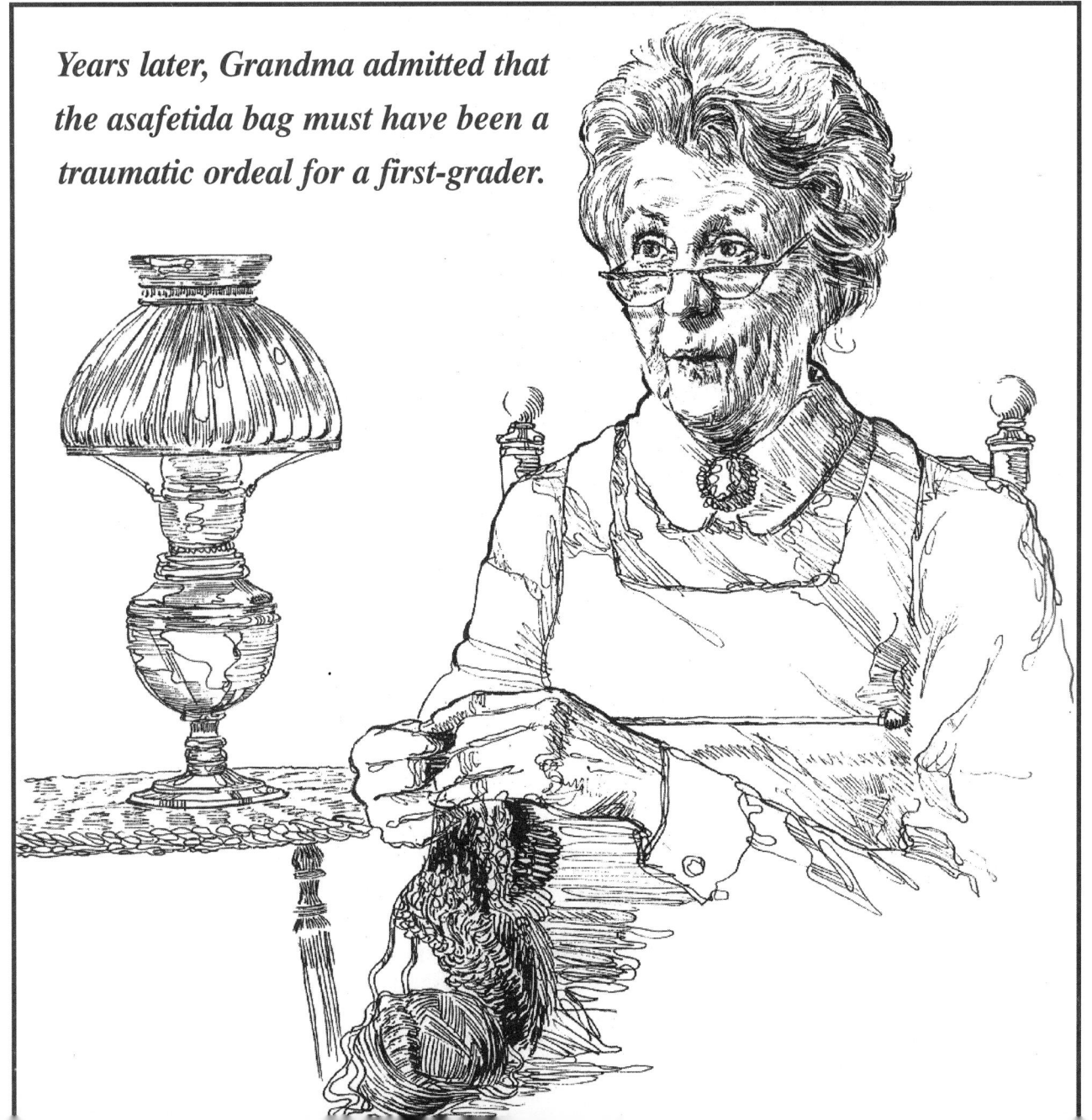

Years later, Grandma admitted that the asafetida bag must have been a traumatic ordeal for a first-grader.

The Doctor Book

By Lee Mann

The Doctor Book contained information about any medical problem Mother had ever heard of, or, God forbid, ever would.

When my mother went to Montana in 1912 to visit her brothers who were homesteading newly opened lands in Wheatland County at the foot of the Rockies, she fell in love with the country. She never really became a Westerner though, being terrified of horses, the wind, the blizzards and the rough-talking natives, but she stayed.

Her father bought her a "relinquishment," a quarter section of land some other homesteader had given up on, and she married the handsome schoolteacher from Oregon who lived on the homestead adjacent to hers. They moved into a three-room shack on Mother's homestead.

Mother retreated temporarily to the safety of her parents' home in civilized Ohio for the birth of her first child, my sister Ruth. On her return to Montana in the winter of 1916, her trunks were packed with a number of things more needed on a homestead than pretty clothes—sacks of dried popcorn, bags of sassafras bark, her smelling salts in a dark green bottle and her Doctor Book.

The Book was huge, four inches thick and covered with rich blue cloth handsomely lettered in gold. It contained information about any medical problem Mother had ever heard of, or, God forbid, ever would. In addition to remedies for illnesses and instructions for diagnosing them, there were recipes for puddings and gravies for invalids, tables of weights and measures, diagrams for cutting up beef, poultry and pork. Most homesteaders had such a book and their children improved their reading skills by poring over the contents on long winter evenings.

Some of the instructions were practical: "Keep gloomy visitors out of the sickroom."

Some doubtful: "Nervous people are greatly benefited by a diet of celery. Onions are next best." Also: "For a felon, dip the finger in boiling water several times in succession. Repeat every hour for several hours."

Some were probably welcomed by men with disapproving wives: "For rattlesnake bite, moisten fresh earth with water or saliva, apply and bind above wound with handkerchief. Send for enough whiskey to

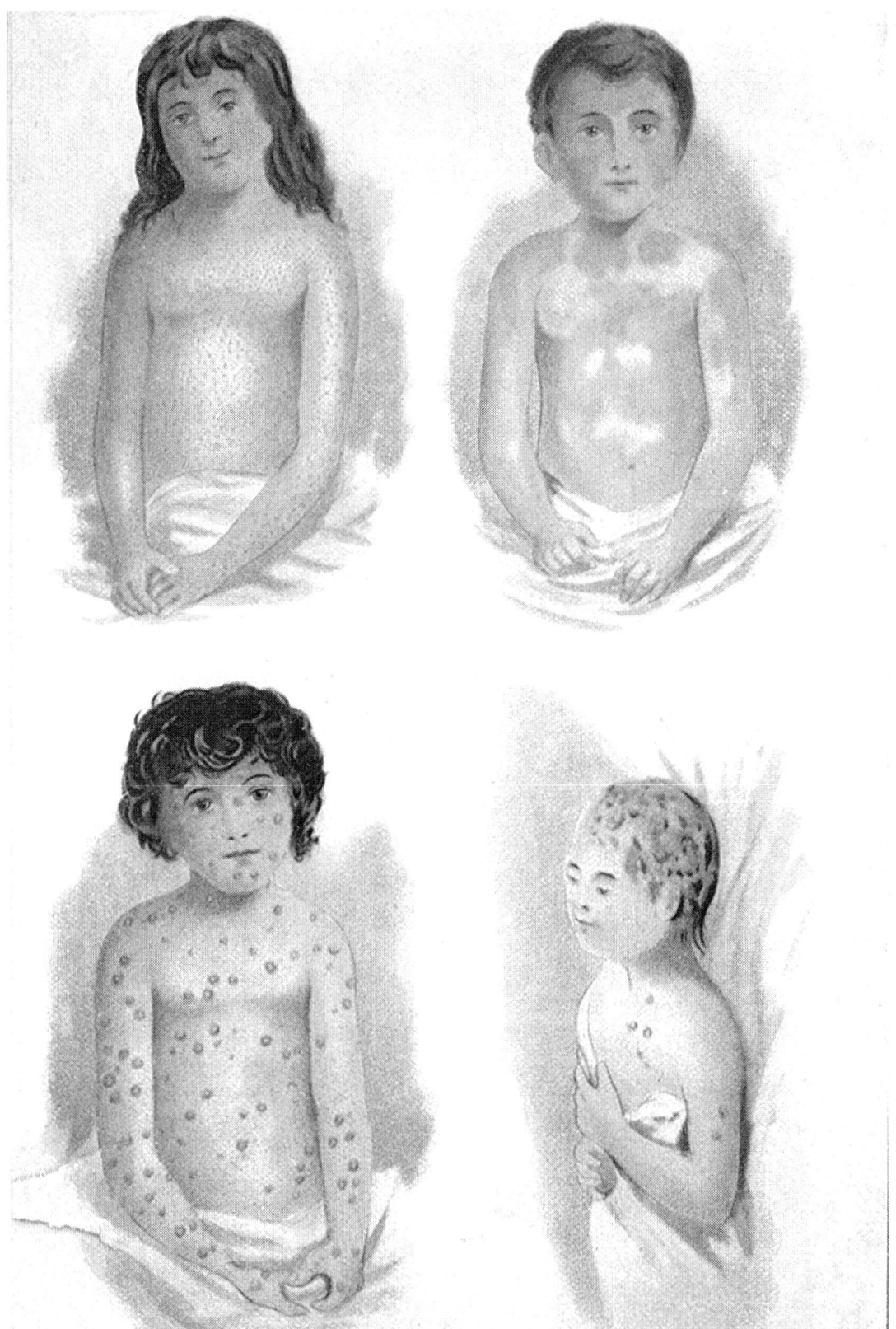

For Treatment of Above See Chapter "Children and Their Diseases."

Fig. 1.   Measles.   Fig. 3.   Scarlet Fever.
Fig. 2.   Chicken Pox.   Fig. 4.   Milk Crust.

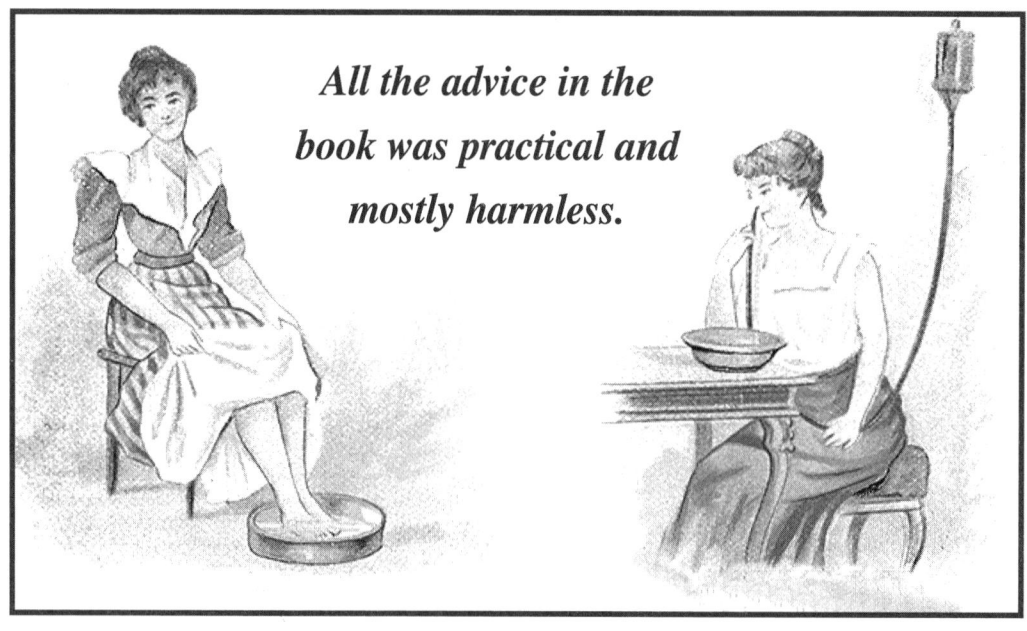

All the advice in the book was practical and mostly harmless.

for a tasty cough syrup made by slicing onions into a heavy white bowl and covering the slices with a generous amount of sugar. The bowl sat in the warming oven of the wood-burning kitchen range until the onion juice and sugar melted into a lovely thick, warm syrup. We could hardly wait for it to get done but we got only a spoonful at a time. After all, it was supposed to be medicine.

completely stupefy him as soon as possible!"

There were real colored photographs of children covered with large or small red blotches, illustrating smallpox, chicken pox, or measles. The size of the spots was a primary clue as to which ailment one had. We escaped smallpox, but both Ruth and I managed to get chicken pox and measles. How remained a mystery, since we were so isolated from neighbors. Nonetheless Doc Campbell was hailed when he passed by on one of the occasional visits he made to his own place several miles from us.

He determined which problem we had—measles—confined us to bed and nailed a quarantine sign on our gate. "Nobody but the cows'll see it, but it's the law," he explained.

Mother had complete faith in her Doctor Book, but she needed products with brand names to carry out the suggested treatment. When we had a cold, our chest and armpits were rubbed with Vicks Vapo-Rub and a bit was stuffed up our noses. If it was a heavy chest cold with fever, we went to bed and were dosed with quinine capsules or worse, Calomel pills. The latter were very small, pale yellow and so bitter they gave one goose bumps.

A sore throat meant gargling with warm salt water and/or wrapping the throat with a towel soaked in cold water. We didn't mind sore throats because there was a recipe in the Book

So was the sassafras tea we often had for supper on winter evenings. Ruth and I were in charge of making it. We put a handful of the dark red chips into a big blue enamel bowl and poured boiling water over it, put on a cover and let the tea steep until it was the right color. We dipped the tea into cups with a soup ladle. With a spoonful of sugar and a dash of real cream, the rosy brew was a treat. It was said to be good for thinning the blood which was not really what was needed where the temperature could and did reach 50 below, but since we didn't know that thicker blood would be more the thing, we felt we got great benefit from the tea.

Intestinal disorders were not so pleasantly prescribed for. Treatment—castor oil, which I never could keep down long enough for any benefit even when the stuff was cut with hot coffee. A simple stomachache was treated with a spoonful of Raleigh's liniment in water, with, of course, a teaspoonful of sugar.

I had frequent earaches, the result of bad tonsils and failure to wear a stocking cap when the wind was howling, and it usually was. Lying in bed with my throbbing ear resting on a bag of warm salt or having a few drops of warm oil poured in never helped so much as did the tobacco smoke from Dad's pipe, puffed gently in while I sat whimpering on his lap.

Once Ruth and I both got ringworm crusts on our hands (from dogs, according to the Book). Following instructions, Mother boiled up a gooey mess of brown sugar and laundry soap and painted the crusts. Not even ringworm could hold out against Mother's laundry soap made from rancid scraps of fat and lye water.

The seven-year itch we brought home from school took longer to cure than anything we got. Mother and Dad got it too. All four of us rubbed nightly most of one winter with a salve made from coal oil and other ingredients. It smelled abominable, but the itch finally disappeared, either cured or worn out.

We had a choice of treatments for cuts from barbed wire or knives, and I'm not sure the Doctor Book suggested any of them. It did say to wash well with soap and water, but we were rarely near soap or water when a gash occurred. Peroxide was handy in the kitchen to fizzle our dirt, but if the wound looked too severe, Mother insisted on iodine. It burned like fury, enough to satisfy the patient that it was doing the job. It may have, but it also caused the nearest to death from treatment I ever suffered.

As a teen-ager I was plagued with acne, and when a big red lump appeared on my chin, I determined to dry it up with a coat of iodine. Instead of disappearing the lump got bigger and began to throb alarmingly. Worse, I became feverish, my head pounded as the swelling spread and within 24 hours I was so ill I lay all day on Mother's bed, sort of going in and out of it. Dad was gone for the day and Mother frequently came in to look thoughtfully at me, but she said nothing to alarm me.

As soon as Dad came home in the evening, he bundled me into the Model T and took me to town to the hospital. Fortunately it was one of the times when the hospital was open for business with a doctor present. He lanced the angry red swelling on my chin and for the first and only time in my life I fainted.

Years later Dad came to Oregon to visit and we did a lot of reminiscing about our homestead days. Dad said, "Remember the time I took you to the hospital to have that abscess lanced? I've thought about that often. You could have died."

I had not thought of that possibility before,

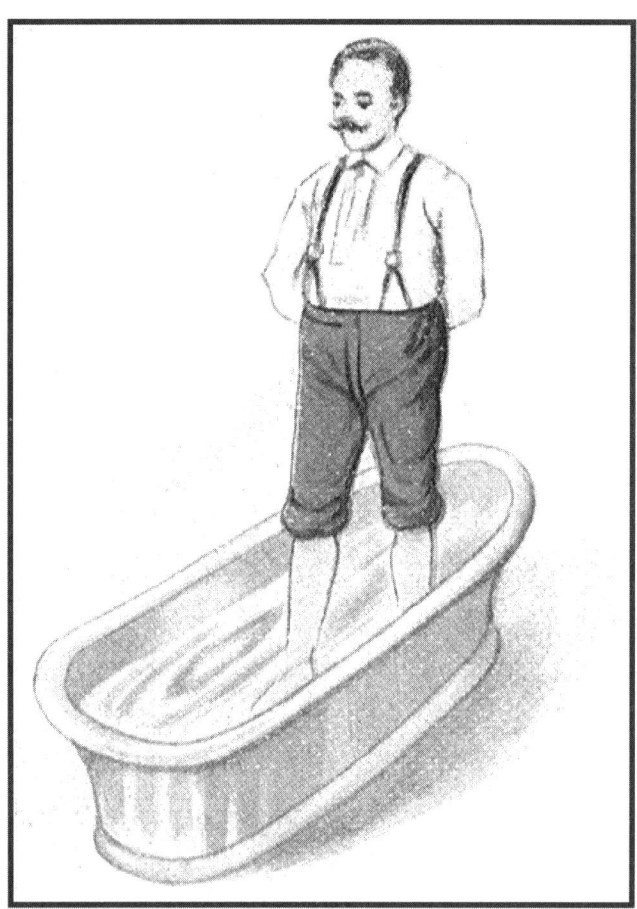

There were real photographs in the book to help in diagnosis.

and it came to me how remarkable it was that so many homesteaders, living miles from any medical help, did survive the primitive treatment available to them. The potential for disaster was always present.

The Book had information on treating animals for cuts and warbles, ridding the house of flies, preserving eggs and making a poultice for boils. We found out how to cure a ham, set a broken bone, make a splint. All the advice was practical and mostly harmless. Materials needed were to be found in any household. After all, you couldn't step out to the drugstore to fill a prescription.

The Book took the place for us of doctor, hospital and psychiatrist. One of the key ingredients for success is having faith in the advisor, and every homesteader had faith in the Doctor Book. He had to—there was no other help at hand in a crisis. ◆

Granny Woman

By Susan L. Bates

My husband's grandmother was a midwife, or "granny woman" as they were called in the Ozark hills. She was the mother of 12 children and had brought every one of them into the world herself!

Grandpa was a sharecropper and he also worked in small sawmills—jobs that offered poor pay and even poorer living conditions.

When one of the children was sick or injured Grandma didn't have the luxury of taking him to the doctor.

If her storehouse of knowledge didn't include the right cure for the problem, she would pray until the answer came to her. What faith!

Through numerous illnesses, snakebites, head wounds and broken bones, Grandma kept her brood alive. She was proud of the fact that she never lost a "young'un."

When her son's young wife went into labor, a doctor was sent for. Hours went by and the girl was in agony.

Grandma was right there, giving her herbs and doing what she knew how to do. Finally it became clear that both mother and child were going to die if something wasn't done.

Grandma discovered that the baby was breech, and went about turning it around. Soon a very sickly blue little boy was born. She cleared his lungs of mucous and blew her own breath into him. When this failed to bring about a cry, she had his new aunts dip him alternately into warm and cold water. He began to cry, weakly at first, but he was alive. Hours later the country doctor showed up drunk.

Sickness was kept at bay with an asafetida bag. Worn around the neck, it contained evil-smelling herbs and potions. Not only did it keep illness away, but most people steered clear too.

As a child my husband, deemed sickly by Grandma, would be attached to a medicine bag at the beginning of the cold and flu season. Of course he couldn't stand to have the thing on and, being a normal child, would take the bag off and hide it every chance he got. He never understood how Grandma could always find it.

Once when she was older, Grandma had a severe pain in her stomach. She went through all of her cures, but the pain just got worse

They knew that when sickness came calling, Grandma could handle it.

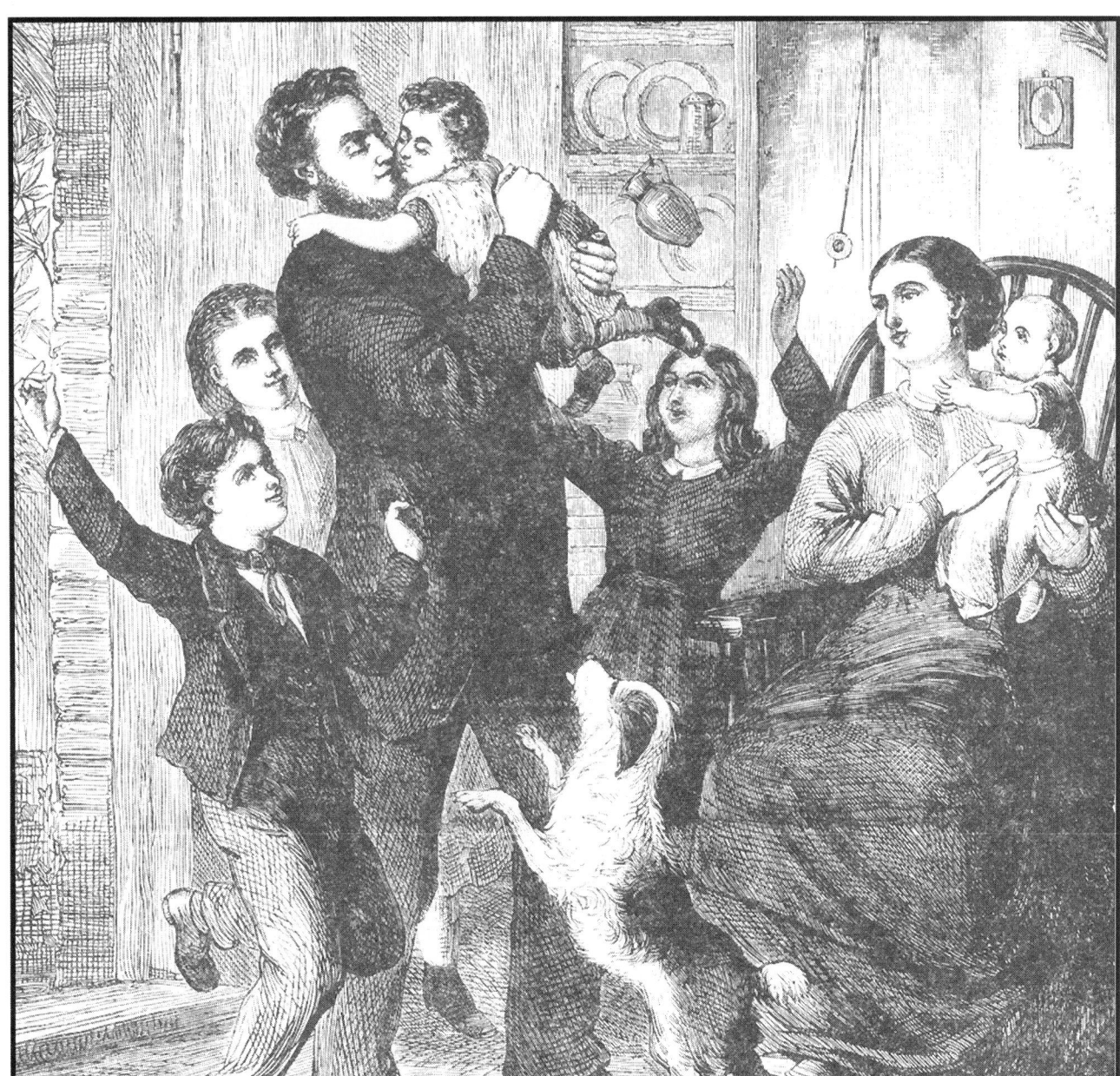

and worse. She thought that she might die. Her daughters persuaded her to go into town and see the doctor. However, this was Saturday night and she would have to last until Monday.

She prayed and prayed for God to tell her what to do. Finally she got up and ate a raw potato. Asked why she was doing that, she just said that the potato would cure her.

By Monday morning the pain had eased quite a bit. Grandma decided that she didn't need to waste money seeing a doctor, but her daughters weren't convinced that eating a potato could do much for a body. Reluctantly, Grandma made the trip to town.

The doctor found that she had an abscess in her stomach. The abscess probably would have killed her before Monday if she hadn't eaten a raw potato to absorb some of the poison.

Grandma raised 12 children, all but two living to old age. Most of the time they didn't have enough to eat, shoes for their feet or warm coats in the winter.

But they knew a mother and father's love. And they knew that when sickness came calling, Grandma could handle it. It is too bad that she didn't write down some of her cures.

That kind of wisdom is more precious than gold. ◆

MEDICATION MEDITATION

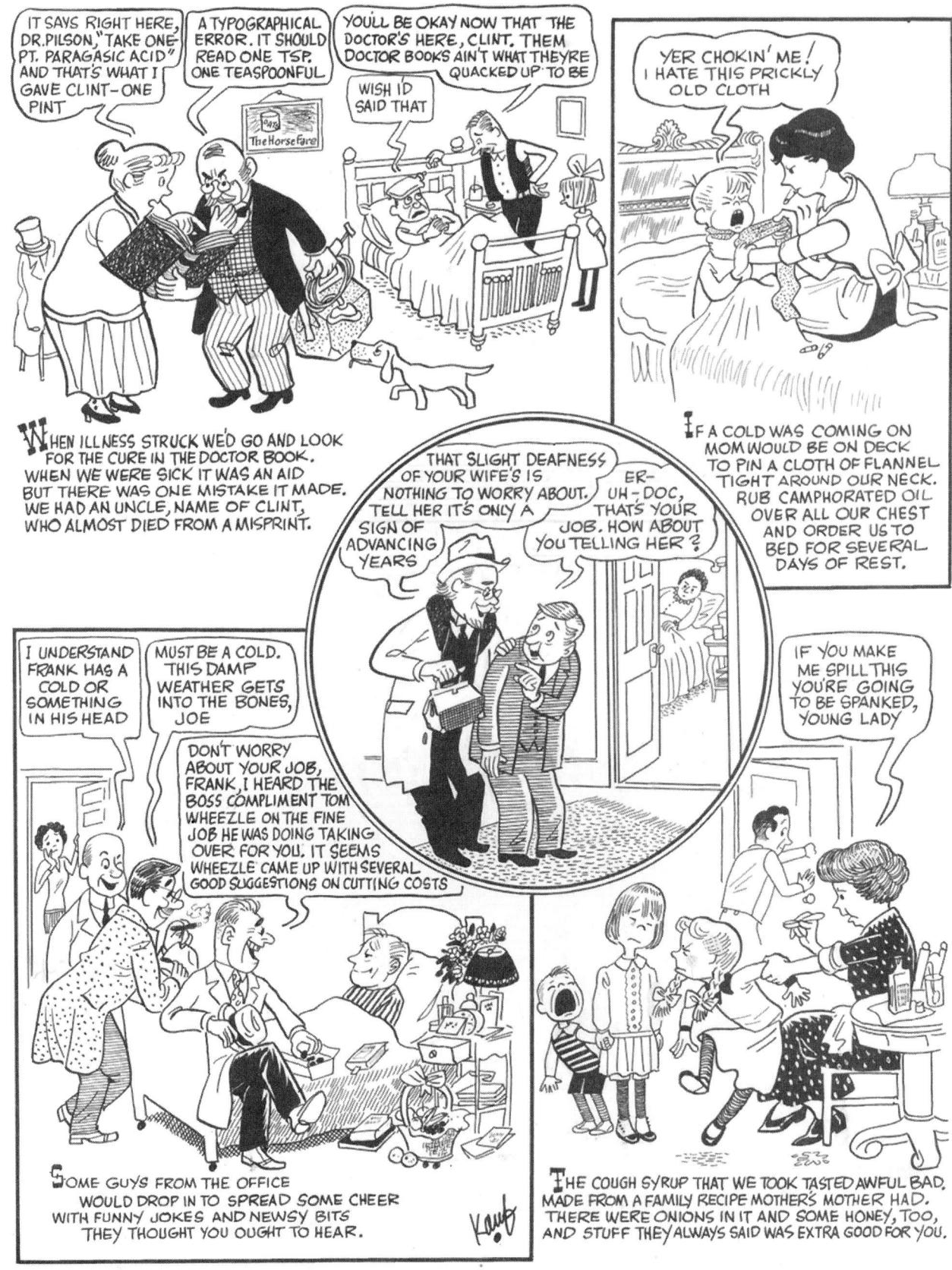